INDIGENOUS PEOPLES
AND DEMENTIA

INDIGENOUS PEOPLES AND DEMENTIA

New Understandings of Memory Loss and Memory Care

Edited by Wendy Hulko,
Danielle Wilson, and
Jean E. Balestrery

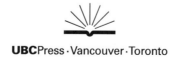

UBCPress · Vancouver · Toronto

27 26 25 24 23 22 21 20 19   5 4 3 2 1

Printed in Canada on FSC-certified ancient-forest-free paper (100% post-consumer recycled) that is processed chlorine- and acid-free.

ISBN 978-0-7748-3783-5 (hardcover)
ISBN 978-0-7748-3784-2 (softcover)
ISBN 978-0-7748-3785-9 (PDF)
ISBN 978-0-7748-3786-6 (EPUB)
ISBN 978-0-7748-3787-3 (Kindle)

Cataloguing data is available from Library and Archives Canada.

Canadä

UBC Press gratefully acknowledges the financial support for our publishing program of the Government of Canada (through the Canada Book Fund), the Canada Council for the Arts, and the British Columbia Arts Council.

Printed and bound in Canada by Friesens
Set in Garamond and Meta Pro by Sharlene Eugenio
Copy editor: Deborah Kerr
Proofreader: Kristy Lynn Hankewitz

UBC Press
The University of British Columbia
2029 West Mall
Vancouver, BC V6T 1Z2
www.ubcpress.ca

CONTENTS

FOREWORD

She: kon.

In 2013, a month before I took up my new position as professor and BC research chair in Indigenous health at Thompson Rivers University, I was invited to a research forum hosted by the editors of this book to discuss and celebrate the results of a project they had recently completed. It explored the subject of Indigenous people and dementia. I was particularly impressed with the way in which the investigators transferred the results of their research in a culturally appropriate and effective way. Five years later, they continue to mobilize their knowledge by editing this valuable volume.

The book provides a good primer on dementia and memory loss as well as some valuable perspectives on how differing worldviews in general, and Indigenous worldviews in particular, can affect our understanding of dementia and memory loss. Because I am one of the few Indigenous mental health psychologists and mental health researchers in Canada, I do not have the luxury of specializing in a single area of mental health because I can't justifiably confine myself to one aspect of mental health. Nor would I want to, as Indigenous health research and practice is holistic in nature and encompasses the mental, physical, emotional, and spiritual. In other words, I know a little bit about a large number of Indigenous health concerns. To the best of my knowledge, this book represents the first significant contribution to what we know about how Indigenous peoples understand dementia and memory loss.

This book is unique in featuring teaching stories. Traditional stories can be interpreted in many ways, and it is up to each listener to determine what they mean to him or her. Several years ago, one of these stories was shared with me, and I have often used it when talking about Indigenous research. As it involves Coyote, failing memory, and research, I thought it appropriate to share with the readers of this book. It was told to me by another Indigenous professor and colleague, Dr. Jo-Ann Archibald (Stó:lō Nation). Jo-Ann received the story from yet another Indigenous professor and colleague, Dr. Eber Hampton (Chickasaw Nation). I hope I have done justice to your story, Jo-Ann and Eber.

> Old Man Coyote was on a long journey and had just finished a hard day of walking. He decided to set up his camp for the night and to have his supper. After supper, he sat by the fire and rubbed his feet, which were tired from the long day's walk. When he looked at his moccasins, he noticed that there was a hole in one of them. He looked for his bone needle to sew the moccasin, but he couldn't find it in his bag. Old Man Coyote started to crawl on his hands and knees on the ground around the fire, hoping to see or feel the needle. Just then, Owl flew over to Coyote and asked him what he was looking for. Old Man explained that he couldn't remember where he put his bone needle. Owl said that he would help Coyote look for it. After he flew around the fire a few times, he told Old Man Coyote that he didn't see the needle and if it was around the fire, he would have spotted it because his night vision was very good. He then asked Old Man Coyote where he last used the needle. Old Man Coyote said that he used it a few days ago, maybe thirty or forty miles north of here, when he had mended a rip in his jacket. Then Owl asked him why he was searching for the needle around the campfire. Old Man Coyote said, "Well, it's much easier to look for the needle here because the fire gives off such good light, and I can see much better here."

Whether you identify with Old Man Coyote, with Owl, or with some other feature of this story, I trust that the light provided by this book will illuminate the tools that will help you with your journey.

Skén:nen – peace

Rod McCormick (Kanienkehaka), professor and
British Columbia Innovation Council research chair
in Aboriginal Health, Faculty of Education and
Social Work, Thompson Rivers University

INDIGENOUS PEOPLES
AND DEMENTIA

INTRODUCTION

Wendy Hulko, Jean E. Balestrery,
and Danielle Wilson

DEMENTIA IS ON THE RISE among non-Indigenous and Indigenous popu-lations around the world.[1] In Canada, approximately half a million people have dementia, and the Alzheimer Society of Canada (2010) reports that this number will more than double over the next thirty years. In the United States, more than 5 million Americans have dementia, and another 15 million have been identified as family caregivers (Lindberg 2014). And even though only approximately 48,000 New Zealanders were living with dementia in 2011, the Ministry of Health reported in 2013 that this number is expected to increase by over 60 percent by 2026.

Dementia has real costs that have prompted action plans by governments around the world. It has been estimated, for instance, that half a million Americans die each year of dementia, resulting in more than $140 billion spent annually in excess Medicare and Medicaid payments by the federal government (Lindberg 2014). A national plan to address dementia came together in 2011, when Congress passed the National Alzheimer's Project Act. This legislation supported the National Alzheimer's Project, one major goal of which was to decrease "disparities in Alzheimer's for ethnic and racial minority populations" and to "coordinate with international bodies to fight Alzheimer's globally" (U.S. Department of Health and Human Services 2014, 3; see also National Quality Forum 2014).

New Zealand's Ministry of Health followed suit in 2013, with its New Zealand Framework for Dementia Care. The framework explicitly acknow-ledged that dementia care must "consider the needs of Maori and other ethnicities" (Ministry of Health 2013, 3). In June 2017, Canada passed its own legislation, becoming the thirtieth country to create a national dementia strategy (Alzheimer Society of Canada 2017).[2] Seven provinces, including Ontario and Quebec, had previously developed and implemented province-wide plans to respond to the projected increase of people with dementia, and the Alzheimer Society of Canada and the Alzheimer Society of B.C. had commissioned a major study, completed by RiskAnalytica in 2009.[3]

This study concluded that system navigators – people or agencies who see the health system as a whole – could reduce the "economic burden of dementia." Unfortunately, it and other social policy studies employed what Anne Robertson (1990) refers to as "apocalyptic demography" to advance their cause.[4] They placed little emphasis on persons with dementia as citizens who had rights to dignity and care (Bartlett and O'Connor 2010) and instead added to the crisis discourse that has made dementia the most feared diagnosis (George and Whitehouse 2014; Whitehouse and George 2008). Though we recognize that rising rates of dementia pose a challenge to provinces, states, and nations, we wrote this book in response to a need – expressed by communities and practitioners – for information on how best to address memory loss and memory care in Indigenous communities in the context of efforts to achieve health equity. For example, a needs assessment conducted by the Alzheimer Society of B.C. in 1998 identified a lack of awareness of dementia and a desire for more information on the part of local First Nations (Alzheimer Society of B.C., Central Interior Region 1998). The New Zealand Framework for Dementia Care (Ministry of Health 2013, 3) recognized that Māori have "a higher rate of risk factors for dementia" than other New Zealanders. In Ontario, Indigenous health organizations began to report an increase in dementia in their communities in 2007 (Sutherland 2007). These demands for information coalesced with the United Nations Declaration on the Rights of Indigenous Peoples, which states that "Indigenous individuals have an equal right to the enjoyment of the highest attainable standard of physical and mental health" (United Nations 2007, Article 24.2). The product of more than thirty years of activism by the global Indigenous movement, the declaration aims to ameliorate health disparities among Indigenous peoples around the world.

Although dementia in Indigenous populations is a relatively new area of research, the rates have been increasing among Indigenous people every-where. And we know that the types and causes of dementia in Indigenous communities differ from those in other populations. Whereas policy makers and service providers have only recently taken up Indigenous people and dementia as an area of concern, epidemiological research on this topic began more than twenty-five years ago, when it was discovered that Alzheimer's was rare among Cree people in Manitoba (Hendrie et al. 1993). Over the next few decades, anthropologists and other social scientists focused their research on the meanings that Indigenous people, particularly Elders, ascribe to memory loss in later life and identified issues related to assessment and care.[5] The contributors to this volume build on this knowledge base and are collectively committed to honouring knowledge translation and Indigenous research methodologies and working in collaboration with Indigenous communities and nations (Kovach 2009; Tuhiwai Smith 2012; Wilson 2008). Most adopt a decolonizing approach and recommend culturally safe care, a stance that reflects the changing landscape of Indigenous health research.

To decolonize something is to call into question the existence and legitimacy of the settler colonial state and to mobilize Indigenous people and their allies to work toward the demise of settler colonialism in all its forms (Simpson and Smith 2014; Tuck and Yang 2012). This means dismantling structures and processes that were put in place to monitor, control, and oppress Indigenous peoples. As Eve Tuck and Wayne Yang (2012, 1) so eloquently put it, decolonization "brings about the repatriation of Indigenous land and life; it is not a metaphor." In the fields of child welfare and health services, decolonization entails devolving responsibility to Indigenous communities, thereby promoting their self-determination. Decolonization is best achieved by working in collaboration, and settlers are integral to the process. Following Tuck and Yang, our definition of "settlers" goes beyond people of white European descent to encompass racialized people, including those from other colonial contexts: "settler colonialism and its decolonization implicates and unsettles everyone" (Tuck and Yang 2012, 7). Decolonization is not simply about returning to the past or romanticizing it but about combining its lessons with current realities (Cardenas Aguilar 2015; see also Hulko et al. 2010).

A decolonizing approach underpins the concept of culturally safe care. Developed by Irapeti Ramsden, a Māori nurse, in 1990, the concept of cultural safety has been adopted by nurses across Canada, particularly those working with Indigenous people, and by other health disciplines, including social work. Researchers and practitioners of culturally safe care acknowledge the power imbalances that are inherent in relationships between service providers and service users, and they shift the power toward the latter. They recognize cultural safety as both a process and an outcome of giving and receiving care or doing research in collaboration with Indigenous people.[6]

Our research is grounded in the knowledge translation and exchange paradigm, a critical framework for collaborative research.[7] The Canadian Institutes of Health Research (CIHR 2012, 1) defines knowledge translation as "a dynamic and iterative process that includes synthesis, dissemination, exchange and ethically sound application of knowledge to improve the health of Canadians, provide more effective health services and products and strengthen the health care system." Since 2005, networks have formed to foster dementia knowledge transfer – with its emphasis on "partnership and multidirectional communication" to address changing or varied definitions of dementia – at the local, national, and international levels (Illes, Chahal, and Beattie 2011). These include the Alzheimer Knowledge Exchange in Ontario, Canadian Dementia Knowledge Translation Network, a US-based coalition called Leaders Engaged in Alzheimer's Disease, and the International Indigenous Dementia Research Network; the membership of the latter encompasses researchers and decision makers from across Canada, the United States, New Zealand, and Australia, many of whom contributed to this book.

However, as Janet Smylie, Michelle Olding, and Carolyn Ziegler point out in "Sharing What We Know about Living a Good Life: Indigenous Approaches to Knowledge Translation" (2014), the CIHR definition of knowledge does not recognize that "knowing" and "doing" are intertwined and indistinguishable in Indigenous knowledge systems. Intended to en-courage Canadian heath researchers to take up the knowledge translation challenge, the definition fails to suggest that Indigenous knowledge trans-lation strategies and protocols are "dynamic, participatory, integrated into family and community activities, repeated or cyclical, and intergenerational" (Smylie, Olding, and Ziegler 2014, 18). They should be pursued and adhered to throughout the research process, not merely at the end of a project.

We recognize that relationship-centred care and other recent approaches to dementia care that emphasize family and community involvement align more closely with Indigenous principles than does person-centred care; however, the latter is still "considered the gold standard" by the Institutes of Medicine (World Health Organization and Alzheimer's Disease International 2012). The person-centred approach recognizes the inherent dignity of the person living with dementia – that is, that they are a person first – and strives to limit ill-being and maximize well-being in dementia care (Kitwood 1997; Love and Pinkowitz 2013). But its Eurocentric focus on and lionization of the individual may not align well with Indigenous approaches to Elder care. Individuality stands in sharp contrast to Indigenous principles of relationality and interconnectedness (see Hulko and Stern 2009; Jenkins 2014).

Although the contributions to this volume are grounded in the knowledge translation and exchange paradigm, we emphasize that research and practice should ultimately be shaped by Indigenous worldviews rather than by the simplistic application of models of dementia care to Indigenous people. As Leroy Little Bear (2000, 77) succinctly states, "one of the problems with colonialism is that it tries to maintain a singular social order by means of force and law, suppressing the diversity of human worldviews." For Indigenous people, energy is central to life, and the world is in constant motion. This belief underpins a holistic and cyclical view of the world, which is encapsulated in the medicine wheel and the circle of life. Though some scholars (see Hart 2009, 35) assert that Indigenous cultures share certain core concepts such as wholeness, balance, harmony, growth, and healing, Little Bear emphasizes that Indigenous worldviews are always firmly rooted in a particular place. The concept of relationality – one's connection to land and space and all that lives on and within it – is integral to Indigenous worldviews and explains why many Elders refer to "all my relations" when they pray to the Creator (Hulko 2014, 97).

Indigenous worldviews have only recently been taken into account in the naming and diagnosis of dementia and Alzheimer's disease. The umbrella term "dementia" applies to various forms of cognitive impairment that affect mostly older adults, the primary symptoms of which are memory loss, word-finding difficulties, disorientation, and impaired judgment (Alzheimer Society of Canada 2015). Alzheimer's disease is a specific type of dementia, which was identified by Alois Alzheimer in 1906. Except for the genetic type of Alzheimer's, the disease can be conclusively diagnosed solely by the postmortem identification of the plaques and tangles that it produces in the brain. Dementia is predominantly associated with older people today, and the word itself is often used interchangeably with Alzheimer's disease in everyday discourse. But there is a case for avoiding it altogether. In many ethnocultural and Indigenous communities, the word may not exist or hold any meaning in their language, or it may have uniformly negative connotations. Secwepemc Elders recommend using "memory loss" and "memory care" (Hulko et al. 2010). We recognize that these terms privilege memory and its loss over other symptoms of dementia, but memory loss is the hallmark of dementia and perhaps a more easily recognizable feature of impaired cognition than disorientation or language difficulties, for example. And, as Barbara Purves and Wendy Hulko demonstrate in Chapter 8 of this volume, memory holds special meaning for Indigenous people.

Indigenous worldviews have likewise influenced diagnosis. The diagnosis of dementia – by a physician or a psychiatrist, in a doctor's office or a memory clinic – often involves the Mini-Mental State Examination (see Beard 2016). However, this test has been criticized for being a culturally relative (and hence unreliable) assessment tool. Researchers and clinicians have sought to develop "culture fair" alternatives that can enable more accurate diagnoses of cognitive impairment in certain ethnocultural groups. For Indigenous people, these tools include the Kimberley Indigenous Cognitive Assessment (KICA), created for use in the Kimberley region and the Northern Territory of Australia; the Grasshoppers and Geese test, developed for Cree people in Saskatchewan; and the Canadian Indigenous Cognitive Assessment, adapted from the KICA by Ontario researchers.[8] A key feature of these new screening protocols and assessment tools is the incorporation of visual images that reflect the culture and territory of the person being assessed. They are welcome additions to the clinician's diagnostic skill set, but we need more tools that reflect the uniqueness of Indigenous people. The developers of the KICA note that "Indigenous people are heterogeneous and there is a need to trial tools with people from different areas, language groups, ages and levels of cognitive impairment" (Smith et al. 2007, 118).

With these new approaches and methods in mind, *Indigenous Peoples and Dementia* opens with "We Call It Healing." This is one of two stories (the other being "Coyote: Keeper of Memories") crafted during a story creation workshop for the Culturally Safe Dementia Care (CSDC) project conducted in collaboration with Elders of the Secwepemc Nation (see Hulko et al. 2014). Secwepemc people traditionally used stories to teach future generations about their environment, social structures, and beliefs, but there are no stories about memory loss or memory care in existence (Hulko et al. 2010). As a team, the workshop participants created new stories originating from community-based research with Secwepemc Elders. Jean William, Cecilia Dick DeRose, and Estella Patrick Moller are the keepers of this new knowledge, and the stories appear in this book with the permission of the CSDC Elders. "We Call It Healing," "Coyote: Keeper of Memories," and a third story or teaching interlude, "A Fecund Frontier" (not connected to the workshop), set the stage for the thematic discussions in the volume's three parts by demonstrating how working and researching in collaboration with Indigenous people and communities can be embodied within a knowledge translation and exchange framework. These stories teach us that the act of sharing – whether it be personal experience or traditional values or while working together – requires deep listening. The Secwepemc Elder in "We Call It Healing" imparts an important lesson for us all: "The past carries forward into the future," and "If the emotional bruises are healed – through sweats, smudging, love, and the Creator – then the dementia can be healed or the impact of living with it lessened." The Coyote story similarly showcases storytelling as medicine among Indigenous people and a powerful way to pass traditional values, principles of living, and knowledge about memory loss and memory care to future generations. The final story, "A Fecund Frontier," by Jean Balestrery and Sophie "Eqeelana Tungwenuk" Nothstine, reveals the productive possibilities for colearning that can emerge when two people of differing worldviews and cultural backgrounds come together.

Part 1, "Prevalence, Causes, and Public Discourse," includes three chapters that directly address the complexities of memory loss and dementia in Indigenous communities. We know that prevalence rates vary from community to community and are trending upward, but we do not fully understand why. For example, dementia is on the rise among First Nations people in British Columbia due to the aging of the Indigenous population in Canada and the prevalence of risk factors linked to colonization such as obesity, diabetes, poverty or low socioeconomic status, low levels of formal education, and cardiovascular disease (British Columbia Provincial Health Officer 2009). Risk factors, which vary from population to population, are generally categorized as modifiable or non-modifiable. The former include external causes such as lifestyle, place of residence, and income. The latter, which cannot be altered, include genetic or hereditary traits. As the BC example suggests, Indigenous people, as an oppressed group, often experience numerous modifiable risk factors that are barriers to health equity and services (Greenwood et al. 2015). Hereditary factors are less common among Indigenous populations than non-Indigenous ones, and to date, only two families are known to have been diagnosed with early onset familial Alzheimer's in Canada (B. Butler et al. 2010; B. Lynn Beattie, pers. comm., August 2010).

In Chapter 1, Jennifer Walker and Kristen Jacklin discuss current and projected rates of dementia prevalence in Canada, noting that the demographic pressures and risk factors encountered by most Indigenous populations are similar to those for First Nations in British Columbia. In Chapter 2, Neil Henderson, Linda Carson, and Kama King continue the discussion by exploring modifiable and non-modifiable risk factors and by proposing what they call an Indigenous Syndemic Dementia Model. The section concludes with Suzanne MacLeod's "A Story about Joe in the News Media," a fascinating analysis of the "crisis" discourse that prevails in contemporary media accounts of persons with dementia. MacLeod argues that these news stories represent ongoing colonizing practices because they cast the Indigenous person as dangerous and the white person as an innocent victim. They are devoid of history and context.

Part 2, "Indigenous Perspectives on Care and Prevention," includes three chapters that bring lived experiences, traditional knowledge, and community insights to bear on memory loss and memory care. Recognizing that the language of biomedicine does not resonate well with many Anishinaabe people, Jessica Pace and her colleagues explore Anishinaabe traditional knowledge about dementia prevention by using the medicine wheel. Similarly, in Chapter 5, Carrie Bourassa and her colleagues employ Indigenous research methods and draw on interviews and focus groups with Indigenous caregivers to delineate the unique challenges of caring for persons with dementia in an Indigenous context. They also make recommendations for support services that foster culturally safe care. In Chapter 6, Mere Kēpa presents a Māori view on aging and memory loss and advocates for whānau-based care, a humanizing form of care centred on Māori principles.

Part 3, "Applying Theory and Knowledge to Practice," focuses explicitly on the application of research to practice. In Chapter 7, Linda Carson, Neil Henderson, and Kama King apply their Indigenous Syndemic Dementia Model to depression and diabetes, highlighting the need to historicize and contextualize these chronic health conditions in order to develop more culturally relevant and safe treatments. In Chapter 8, Barbara Purves and Wendy Hulko explore representations of Indigenous people in a computer-based reminiscence program and its usability with Elders. They argue that we need to proceed cautiously when we use visual imagery that refers to painful historical events. But we should not sanitize the past. Finally, Wendy Hulko, Jessica Kent, and Danielle Wilson reveal what happened when a knowledge translation and exchange framework was applied to the development and evaluation of a storybook and a video for children and youth of the Secwepemc Nation. Incorporating traditional Secwepemc views on aging, the authors produced the book and the film through iterative cycles of community engagement. This method and their evaluation of it indicates that these learning tools can strengthen intergenerational relationships and understanding of memory loss and memory care from a Secwepemc perspective.

Indigenous Peoples and Dementia presents the current state of knowledge on Indigenous people and dementia within a decolonization framework. Our volume promotes culturally safe research and care as settler colonial states and Indigenous communities move toward health equity. Given the recent push for early diagnosis and treatment in dementia care, we need to ask whether this is – or should be – "best practice" with Indigenous people, given their differing worldviews and focus on holism and interconnectedness. Indigenous communities are grappling with tough questions: Is the current (biomedical) approach to dementia at odds with a more holistic view of and response to memory loss in later life? If it is, which approach should we follow, or should we try to reconcile the differences? What does this ultimately mean for Elders living with dementia?[9] We hope that this book provides guidance for nations and communities as they determine the way forward.

As we pass through life, multiple factors influence our physical, spiritual, mental, and emotional health and well-being. Indigenous people throughout Turtle Island share a collective history of oppression, but they also share a history of resilience. This book explores the causal links between this history of oppression and health outcomes such as dementia. Its authors and the researchers – Indigenous people and their allies – contribute new knowledge, or new "cultural narratives" (Zeilig 2014), in support of calls for action to promote and improve dementia-related health outcomes for Elders. Elders are the knowledge keepers of this generation and the valued members of a declining cohort, yet they and their health needs have received little attention in academic research or public policy (Rosenberg et al. 2010). Any measure to protect their health is a step toward rectifying health inequities to better serve generations to come.

Notes

1 Depending on the chapter and context, this volume uses "First Nations," "Aboriginal," "Indigenous," "Indian," and "Native." The terminology differs from country to country and is usually as defined by the first peoples who live there (see Yellow Bird 1999). For instance, in Canada, "First Nations" applies to the first peoples, whereas "Aboriginal" refers to all persons of Indigenous ancestry, including First Nations, Inuit, and Métis. Indigenous people are increasingly expressing the desire to be identified by their specific nation or community and caution against pan-indigenizing (see Kovach 2009). Further, we use "Elder" to refer to all older Indigenous peoples, not only those who serve as traditional knowledge keepers. This is consistent with current practice in Indigenous communities and indicates respect for older community members.

2 This national strategy was announced after our contributors had written their chapters.

3 Ontario's strategy, developed in 1999, comprised ten initiatives to be funded and implemented over a five-year period (McAiney 2005; Ontario Ministry of Health 2015).

4 Similarly, Charlotte Arbogast, E. Ayn Welleford, and Ellen Netting (2017, 840) found "dire prognostications about the progressive and fatal consequences of the disease with a primary focus on the cost" in thirty-eight state dementia plans in the United States. The words "burden" and "crisis" were frequently employed to describe the impact on the state.

5 On Indigenous perceptions of memory loss and approaches to caregiving in the United States, Canada, and Australia, see Browne et al. (2016); Cammer (2006); Finkelstein, Forbes, and Richmond (2012); Forbes et al. (2013); Garvey et al. (2011); J.N. Henderson (2002); J.N. Henderson et al. (2002); S. Henderson and Broe (2010); J.N. Henderson and Carson Henderson (2002); Hulko (2014); Hulko et al. (2010); Hulko et al. (2014); Hulko and Stern (2009); Jacklin and Warry (2012); Jervis and Manson (2002, 2007); Lanting et al. (2011); Lindeman et al. (2012); LoGiudice et al. (2006); O'Connor, Phinney, and Hulko (2010); Jacklin, Pace, and Warry (2015); Pollitt (1997); Smith et al. (2008); Smith et al. (2009); Smith et al. (2011); and Taylor et al. (2012). On early onset familial Alzheimer's disease, see R. Butler et al. (2011) and Stevenson et al. (2013). On risk and prevalence, see Jacklin, Walker, and Shawande (2013). Research in New Zealand with Māori people is still in its early stages, perhaps because it has been more Indigenous-led and/or collaborative there than in Australia. See, for example, the proposal by a Māori and a Pākehā (settler) that a bicultural model be adopted (Martin and Paki 2012).

6 See Aboriginal Nurses Association of Canada (2009); Brascoupé and Waters (2009); Clark et al. (2010); Hulko and Stern (2009); National Aboriginal Health Organization (2008); Ramsden (2005); Smye and Browne (2002); and Wepa (2005).

7 See Estey, Kmetic, and Reading (2008); Smylie et al. (2004); and Smylie, Olding, and Ziegler (2014).

8 See Lanting (2011); LoGiudice et al. (2006); and Pitawanakwat et al. (2016).

9   We thank one of the anonymous peer reviewers for posing thoughtful questions, which we adapted for inclusion herein. We expect they will be answered in time, perhaps in various ways.

References

Aboriginal Nurses Association of Canada. 2009. *Cultural Competence and Cultural Safety in Nursing Education: A Framework for First Nations, Inuit and Métis Nursing.* Ottawa: Aboriginal Nurses Association of Canada. https://www.cna-aiic.ca/~/media/cna/ page-content/pdf-en/first_nations_framework_e.pdf.

Alzheimer Society of B.C., Central Interior Region. 1998, June. *Williams Lake Multicultural Community Assessment Project Summary.* Kamloops, BC: Alzheimer Society of B.C., Central Interior Region.

Alzheimer Society of Canada. 2010. "Rising Tide: The Impact of Dementia on Canadian Society." http://alzheimer.ca/sites/default/files/files/chapters-on/york/rising_tide_ full_report_eng_final.pdf.

–. 2015. "About Dementia." http://www.alzheimer.ca/en/About-dementia.

–. 2017, July 4. "Canada's National Dementia Strategy." http://www.alzheimer.ca/en/ Get-involved/Advocacy/National-dementia-strategy?gclid=EAIaIQobChMI64yH 56zB1gIVklx-Ch1fPQQvEAAYASAAEgJDpfD_BwE.

Arbogast, Charlotte E., E. Ayn Welleford, and F. Ellen Netting. 2017. "State Dementia Plans and the Alzheimer's Disease Movement: Framing Diagnosis, Prognosis, and Motivation." *Journal of Applied Gerontology* 36 (7): 840–63. DOI:10.1177/0733464 815602112.

Bartlett, Ruth, and Deborah O'Connor. 2010. *Broadening the Dementia Debate: Towards Social Citizenship.* Bristol: Policy Press.

Beard, Renee L. 2016. *Living with Alzheimer's: Managing Memory Loss, Identity and Illness.* New York: New York University Press.

Brascoupé, Simon, and Catherine Waters. 2009. "Cultural Safety: Exploring the Applicability of the Concept of Cultural Safety to Aboriginal Health and Community Wellness." *International Journal of Aboriginal Health* 5 (2): 6–41.

British Columbia Provincial Health Officer. 2009. *Pathways to Health and Healing – 2nd Report on the Health and Well-Being of Aboriginal People in British Columbia. Provincial Health Officer's Annual Report 2007.* Victoria: Ministry of Healthy Living and Sport.

Browne, C.V., L.S. Ka'opua, L.L. Jervis, R. Alboroto, and M.L. Trockman. 2016. "United States Indigenous Populations and Dementia: Is There a Case for Culture-Based Psychosocial Interventions?" *Gerontologist* 57 (6): 1–9. DOI:10.1093/geront/gnw059.

Butler, B., B.L. Beattie, U. PuangThong, E. Dwosh, C. Guimond, H. Feldman, G.Y.R. Hsiung, E. Rogaeva, P. St. George Hyslop, and A.D. Sadovnick. 2010. "A Novel PS1 Gene Mutation in a Large Aboriginal Kindred." *Canadian Journal of Neurological Sciences* 37 (3): 359–64.

Butler, R., E. Dwosh, B.L. Beattie, C. Guimond, S. Lombera, E. Brief, J. Illes, and

A.D. Sadovnick. 2011. "Genetic Counseling for Early-Onset Familial Alzheimer Disease in Large Aboriginal Kindred from a Remote Community in British Columbia: Unique Challenges and Possible Solutions." *Journal of Genetic Counselling* 20: 136–42. DOI:10.1007/s10897-010-9334-9.

Cammer, Allison Lee. 2006. "Negotiating Culturally Incongruent Healthcare Systems: The Process of Accessing Dementia Care in Northern Saskatchewan." Master's thesis, University of Saskatchewan.

Cardenas Aguilar, F. 2015, May 31. "Decolonizing Education from Indigenous Perspectives: Constructing a Multidimensional Justice." Keynote lecture at Canadian Society for the Study of Education conference, Ottawa.

CIHR (Canadian Institutes of Health Research). 2012. *Guide to Knowledge Translation Planning at CIHR: Integrated and End of Grant Approaches.* Ottawa: CIHR.

Clark, Natalie, Julie Drolet, Nadine Mathews, Patrick Walton, Paul Tamburro, Jann Derrick, Vicki Michaud, Joanne Armstrong, and Mike Arnouse. 2010. "Decolonizing Field Education: 'Melq'ilwiye' Coming Together: An Exploratory Study in the Interior of Rural British Columbia." *Critical Social Work* 11 (1): 6–25.

Estey, E., A. Kmetic, and J. Reading. 2008. "Knowledge Translation in the Context of Aboriginal Health." *Canadian Journal of Nursing Research* 40 (2): 24–39.

Finkelstein, S.A., D.A. Forbes, and C.A. Richmond. 2012. "Formal Dementia Care among First Nations in Southwestern Ontario." *Canadian Journal on Aging* 31 (3): 257–70.

Forbes, D., C. Blake, E. Thiessen, S. Finkelstein, M. Gibson, D.G. Morgan, M. Markle-Reid, and I. Culum. 2013. "Dementia Care Knowledge Sharing within a First Nations Community." *Canadian Journal on Aging* 32 (4): 360–74.

Garvey, G., D. Simmonds, V. Clements, P. O'Rourke, K. Sullivan, D. Gorman, S. Wise, and E. Beattie. 2011. "Making Sense of Dementia: Understanding amongst Indigenous Australians." *International Journal of Geriatric Psychiatry* 26 (6): 649–56.

George, D.R., and P.J. Whitehouse. 2014. "The War (on Terror) on Alzheimer's." *Dementia* 13 (1): 120–30.

Greenwood, M., S. de Leeuw, N.M. Lindsay, and C. Reading. 2015. *Determinants of Indigenous Peoples' Health in Canada: Beyond the Social.* Toronto: Canadian Scholars Press.

Hart, M.A. 2009. "Anti-colonial Indigenous Social Work: Reflections on an Aboriginal Approach." In *Wícihitowin: Aboriginal Social Work in Canada,* ed. Raven Sinclair, Michael Anthony Hart, and Gord Bruyere, 25–41. Halifax: Fernwood.

Henderson, J. Neil. 2002. "The Experience and Interpretation of Dementia: Cross-Cultural Perspectives." *Journal of Cross-Cultural Gerontology* 17 (3): 195–96.

Henderson, J. Neil, and L. Carson Henderson. 2002. "Cultural Construction of Disease: A 'Supernormal' Construct of Dementia in an American Indian Tribe." *Journal of Cross-Cultural Gerontology* 17 (3): 197–212.

Henderson, J. Neil, R. Crook, J. Crook, J. Hardy, L. Onstead, L. Carson Henderson, P. Mayer, B. Parker, R. Petersen, and B. Williams. 2002. "Apolipoprotein E4 and

Tau Allele Frequencies among Choctaw Indians." *Neuroscience Letters* 324 (1): 77–79.

Henderson, S., and G. Broe. 2010. "Dementia in Aboriginal Australians." *Australian and New Zealand Journal of Psychiatry* 44 (10): 869–71.

Hendrie, H.C., et al. 1993. "Alzheimer's Disease Is Rare in Cree." *International Psychogeriatrics* 5 (1): 5–14.

Hulko, Wendy. 2014. "Digging Up the Roots: Nature and Dementia for First Nation Elders." In *Creating Culturally Appropriate Outside Spaces and Experiences for People with Dementia*, ed. Mary Marshall and Jane Gilliard, 96–104. London: Jessica Kingsley.

Hulko, Wendy, Evelyn Camille, Elisabeth Antifeau, Mike Arnouse, Nicole Bachynksi, and Denise Taylor. 2010. "Views of First Nation Elders on Memory Loss and Memory Care in Later Life." *Journal of Cross-Cultural Gerontology* 25 (4): 317–42. DOI:10.1007/s10823-010-9123-9.

Hulko, Wendy, and Louise Stern. 2009. "Cultural Safety, Decision-Making, and Dementia: Troubling Notions of Autonomy and Personhood." In *Decision Making, Personhood and Dementia: Exploring the Interface*, ed. Deborah O'Connor and Barbara Purves, 70–87. London: Jessica Kingsley.

Hulko, Wendy, Danielle Wilson, Star Mahara, Jean William, Estella Patrick Moller, Cecilia DeRose, Gwen Campbell McArthur, Laura Michel-Evans, and Anna Parkscott. 2014, October. "Culturally Safe Dementia Care: Building the Capacity of Nurses to Care for First Nation Elders with Memory Loss." Workshop presentation at International Network of Indigenous Health Knowledge and Development and Network Environments for Aboriginal Health Research conference, Winnipeg.

Illes, Judy, Neil Chahal, and B. Lynn Beattie. 2011. "A Landscape for Training in Dementia Knowledge Translation (DKT)." *Gerontology and Geriatrics* 32 (3): 260–72.

Jacklin, Kristen, Jessica E. Pace, and Wayne Warry. 2015. "Informal Dementia Caregiving among Indigenous Communities in Ontario, Canada." *Care Management Journals* 16 (2): 106–20. DOI:10.1891/1521-0987.16.2.106.

Jacklin, Kristen M., Jennifer D. Walker, and Marjory Shawande. 2013. "The Emergence of Dementia as a Health Concern among First Nations Populations in Alberta, Canada." *Canadian Journal of Public Health* 104 (1): e39–e44.

Jacklin, Kristen, and Wayne Warry. 2012. "Forgetting and Forgotten: Dementia in Aboriginal Seniors." *Anthropology and Aging Quarterly* 33 (1): 13–21.

Jenkins, Nicholas. 2014. "Dementia and the Inter-Embodied Self." *Social Theory and Health* 12 (2): 125–37.

Jervis, Lori L., and Spero M. Manson. 2002. "American Indians/Alaska Natives and Dementia." *Alzheimer Disease and Associated Disorders* 16 (S2): S89–S95.

–. 2007. "Cognitive Impairment, Psychiatric Disorders, and Problematic Behaviours in a Tribal Nursing Home." *Journal of Aging and Health* 19 (2): 260–74.

Kitwood, T. 1997. *Dementia Reconsidered: The Person Comes First*. Buckingham, UK: Open University Press.

Kovach, Margaret. 2009. *Indigenous Methodologies: Characteristics, Conversations, and Contexts.* Toronto: University of Toronto Press.

Lanting, Shawnda. 2011. "Developing an Assessment Protocol to Detect Cognitive Impairment and Dementia in Cree Aboriginal Seniors and to Investigate Cultural Differences in Cognitive Aging." PhD diss., University of Saskatchewan.

Lanting, Shawnda, Margaret Crossley, Debra Morgan, and Alison Cammer. 2011. "Aboriginal Experiences of Aging and Dementia in a Context of Sociocultural Change: Qualitative Analysis of Key Informant Group Interviews with Aboriginal Seniors." *Journal of Cross-Cultural Gerontology* 26 (1): 103–17.

Lindberg, B.W. 2014. "Policy News: LEAD Coalition Director Discusses Dementia Research Funding Challenges." *Gerontology News,* June, 4–5.

Lindeman, M.A., K.A. Taylor, P. Kuipers, K. Stothers, and K. Piper. 2012. "'We Don't Have Anyone with Dementia Here': A Case for Better Intersectoral Collaboration for Remote Indigenous Clients with Dementia." *Australian Journal of Rural Health* 20 (4): 190–94.

Little Bear, Leroy. 2000. "Jagged Worldviews Colliding." In *Reclaiming Indigenous Voice and Vision,* ed. Marie Battiste, 77–85. Vancouver: UBC Press.

LoGiudice, D., K. Smith, J. Thomas, N.T. Lautenschlager, O.P. Almeida, D. Atkinson, and L. Flicker. 2006. "Kimberley Indigenous Cognitive Assessment Tool (KICA): Development of a Cognitive Assessment Tool for Older Indigenous Australians." *International Psychogeriatrics* 18 (2): 269–80.

Love, K., and J. Pinkowitz. 2013. "Person-Centered Care for People with Dementia: A Theoretical and Conceptual Framework." *GENERATIONS – Journal of the American Society on Aging* 37 (3): 23–29.

Martin, Ros, and Paea Paki. 2012. "Towards Inclusion: The Beginnings of a Bicultural Model of Dementia Care in Aotearoa New Zealand." *Dementia* 11 (4): 545–52. DOI:10.1177/1471301212437821.

McAiney, C. 2005. "The Evaluation of Ontario's Strategy for Alzheimer Disease and Related Dementias: Final Report." https://www.researchgate.net/publication/242714200_The_Evaluation_of_Ontario's_Strategy_for_Alzheimer_Disease_and_Related_Dementias_Final_Report.

Ministry of Health. 2013. *New Zealand Framework for Dementia Care.* Wellington: Ministry of Health.

National Aboriginal Health Organization. 2008, January. *Cultural Competency and Safety: A Guide for Health Care Administrators, Providers and Educators.* Ottawa: National Aboriginal Health Organization.

National Quality Forum. 2014, October 15. "Priority Setting for Healthcare Performance Measurement: Addressing Performance Measure Gaps for Dementia, Including Alzheimer's Disease, Final Report." http://www.qualityforum.org/priority_setting_for_healthcare_performance_measurement_alzheimers_disease.aspx.

O'Connor, Deborah, Alison Phinney, and Wendy Hulko. 2010. "Dementia at the Intersections: A Unique Case Study Exploring Social Location." *Journal of Aging Studies* 24 (1): 30–39. DOI:10.1016/j.jaging.2008.08.001.

Ontario Ministry of Health. 2015. *Ontario's Strategy for Alzheimer Disease and Related Dementias: Preparing for Our Future.* http://www.ontla.on.ca/library/repository/mon/7000/10281575.pdf.

Pitawanakwat, Karen, Kristen Jacklin, Melissa Blind, Megan O'Connell, Wayne Warry, Jennifer Walker, Janet McElhaney, Brock Pitawanakwat, Kate Smith, Dina LoGiudice, and Leon Flicker. 2016. "Adapting the Kimberly Indigenous Cognitive Assessment for Use with Indigenous Older Adults in Canada." *Alzheimer's and Dementia* 12 (7): S311.

Pollitt, P.A. 1997. "The Problem of Dementia in Australian Aboriginal and Torres Strait Islander Communities." *International Journal of Geriatric Psychiatry* 12: 155–63.

Ramsden, Irihapeti. 2005. "Towards Cultural Safety." In *Cultural Safety in Aotearoa, New Zealand,* ed. Dianne Wepa, 2–19. Auckland: Pearson Education New Zealand.

RiskAnalytica. 2009, October. *Rising Tide: The Impact of Dementia in British Columbia, 2008–2038.* Vancouver: Alzheimer Society of B.C.

Robertson, Anne. 1990. "The Politics of Alzheimer's Disease: A Case Study in Apocalyptic Demography." *International Journal of Health Services* 20 (3): 429–42.

Rosenberg, M., K. Wilson, S. Abonyi, K. Beach, and R. Lovelace. 2010. "Older Aboriginal Peoples in Canada: Demographics, Health Status and Access to Health Care." Social and Economic Dimensions of an Aging Population Research Paper No. 240. http://socserv.mcmaster.ca/sedap/p/sedap249.pdf.

Simpson, Audra, and Andrea and Smith, eds. 2014. *Theorizing Native Studies.* Durham, NC: Duke University Press.

Smith, K., L. Flicker, A. Dwyer, G. Marsh, S. Mahajani, O.P. Almeida, N.T. Lautenschlager, D. Atkinson, and D. LoGiudice. 2009. "Assessing Cognitive Impairment in Indigenous Australians – Re-evaluation of the Kimberley Indigenous Cognitive Assessment (KICA) in Western Australia and the Northern Territory." *Australian Psychologist* 44: 54–61.

Smith, K., L. Flicker, N.T. Lautenschlager, O.P. Almeida, D. Atkinson, A. Dwyer, and D. LoGiudice. 2008. "High Prevalence of Dementia and Cognitive Impairment in Indigenous Australians." *Neurology* 71: 1470–73.

Smith, K., L. Flicker, G. Shadforth, E. Carroll, N. Ralph, D. Atkinson, M. Lindeman, F. Schaper, N.T. Lautenschlager, and D. LoGiudice. 2011. "'Gotta Be Sit Down and Worked Out Together': Views of Aboriginal Caregivers and Service Providers on Ways to Improve Dementia Care for Aboriginal Australians." *Rural and Remote Health* 11 (2): 1–14.

Smith, K., D. LoGiudice, A. Dwyer, J. Thomas, L. Flicker, N.T. Lautenschlager, O.P. Almeida, and D. Atkinson. 2007. "'Ngana Minyarti? What Is This?' Development of Cognitive Questions for the Kimberley Indigenous Cognitive Assessment." *Australasian Journal on Ageing* 26: 115–19.

Smye, Vicki, and Annette Browne. 2002. "'Cultural Safety' and the Analysis of Health Policy Affecting Aboriginal People." *Nurse Researcher* 9 (3): 42–56.

Smylie, Janet, C.M. Martin, N. Kaplan-Myrth, L. Steele, C. Tait, and W. Hogg. 2004. "Knowledge Translation and Indigenous Knowledge." *International Journal of Circumpolar Health* 63 (suppl. 2): 139–43.

Smylie, Janet, Michelle Olding, and Carolyn Ziegler. 2014. "Sharing What We Know about Living a Good Life: Indigenous Approaches to Knowledge Translation." *Journal of the Canadian Health Libraries Association/Journal de l'association des bibliothèques de la santé du Canada* 35: 16–23. DOI:10.5596/c14-009.

Stevenson, Shaun, B. Lynn Beattie, Richard Vedan, Emily Dwosh, Lindsay Bruce, and Judy Illes. 2013. "Neuroethics, Confidentiality, and a Cultural Imperative in Early Onset Alzheimer Disease: A Case Study with a First Nation Population." *Philosophy, Ethics, and Humanities in Medicine* 8 (15): 1–6.

Sutherland, M.E. 2007, March. "Alzheimer's Disease and Related Dementias (ADRD) in Aboriginal Communities: New Visions and Understandings." Paper presented at Alzheimer's Disease and Related Dementias within Aboriginal Individuals – Roundtable Forum, Sudbury, ON.

Taylor, K.A., M.A. Lindeman, K. Stothers, K. Piper, and P. Kuipers. 2012. "Intercultural Communications in Remote Aboriginal Australian Communities: What Works in Dementia Education and Management?" *Health Sociology Review* 21 (2): 208–19.

Tuck, Eve, and K. Wayne Yang. 2012. "Decolonization Is Not a Metaphor." *Decolonization: Indigeneity, Education and Society* 1 (1): 1–40. http://decolonization.org/index.php/des/article/view/18630.

Tuhiwai Smith, Linda. 2012. *Decolonizing Methodologies: Research and Indigenous Peoples.* 2nd ed. London: Zed Books.

United Nations. 2007. "The United Nations Declaration on the Rights of Indigenous Peoples (UNDRIP)." http://www.un.org/esa/socdev/unpfii/documents/DRIPS_en.pdf.

U.S. Department of Health and Human Services. 2014. "National Plan to Address Alzheimer's Disease: 2014 Update." Washington, DC, U.S. Department of Health and Human Services. http://aspe.hhs.gov/daltcp/napa/NatlPlan2014.shtml.

Wepa, Dianne, ed. 2005. *Cultural Safety in Aotearoa, New Zealand.* Auckland: Pearson Education New Zealand.

Whitehouse, Peter, with Daniel George. 2008. *The Myth of Alzheimer's: What You Aren't Being Told about Today's Most Dreaded Diagnosis.* New York: St. Martin's Press.

Wilson, Shaun. 2008. *Research Is Ceremony: Indigenous Research Methods.* Halifax: Fernwood.

World Health Organization and Alzheimer's Disease International. 2012. *Dementia: A Public Health Priority.* Geneva: World Health Organization.

Yellow Bird, Michael. 1999. "What We Want to Be Called: Indigenous Peoples' Perspectives on Racial and Ethnic Identity Labels." *American Indian Quarterly* 23 (2): 1–21.

Zeilig, H. 2014. "Dementia as a Cultural Metaphor." *Gerontologist* 54 (2): 258–67.

WE CALL IT HEALING

Secwepemc Elder, Wendy Hulko, Danielle Wilson, Star Mahara, Gwen Campbell-McArthur, Jean William, Cecilia DeRose, and Estella Patrick Moller

This teaching story was narrated by an Elder of the Secwepemc Nation, who wishes to be anonymous.

There Was a Young Boy

》 There was a young boy standing at a window in a classroom, crying his heart out because Mom and Dad had left him there. He wondered why Mom and Dad were doing this. Fear overtook him. And he looked up and seen one of these men in black robes. Then he said, "Who are these people? What am I doing here? Why can't I be with my mom and dad and grandma and grandpa? I miss my dog. Me and Muxie, we used to go and run and play – my dog and I. Muxie would run and catch the pheasants that Dad shot down with his shotgun. Now, this is all gone – including hunting and fishing with my dad. Fishing was my favourite. Oh what will happen to me? I'm like a wolf with nobody with me, all separate from my pack."

The next day he got up from this strange bed, with all kinds of other young boys sleeping around him.

> *I seen so many sad faces. Some of the older boys were talking. "Ha, ha," they laughed, "you gotta get your hair cut." I absolutely froze and said nobody is going to cut my long hair.*

*In the Indian school, I also got kicked, slapped, and
punched for speaking my language. I grew up
ashamed to be an Indian. Years later as I got older
and bigger, I tried to run away from this school. They
would catch me and bring me back, and would I ever
get a strapping. Finally, I left that place a few years
later, and I went to the white man's school where it
was very common to be called a "half-breed bastard"
by my teacher and some of the other students. They
used to say, "sticks and stones will break my bones,
but names will never hurt me," but that's crap – the
names did hurt us. I got to admit one thing about the
Indian school, though it was very painful, they taught
me how to read and write. But I wouldn't recommend
anyone bring their kids there now that I'm an Elder.*

Now That I'm an Elder

>> Now that I'm an Elder, I've been asked to tell my story so as to help with
the care of Elders in senior citizens' homes. Going to Indian residential
school – other than learning how to read and write – has been a very
negative contribution to my health and well-being. I suffered from
alcoholism and tons of fear. And now that we're working on this project
about dementia, it is so important for the nurses and doctors to treat us
with tender loving care because we are so sensitive about the past. We
are learning how to heal, thanks to other loving, healing people. Just by
expressing myself, the healing process is working. And how you use this
story could help others. Finally, I'm not alone. I've got a lot of wonderful
people, helping and supporting me. Thanks to the Creator.

One thing that I'm concerned about if I ever go into a care home is that
they – the nurses and the doctors – will force me to give up my traditional
ways that are so dear and close to me. For example, if I want deer meat,
moose meat, elk, salmon, then I should be allowed to receive this food
from my relatives and friends, and also we should still get herbal
medicines from the naturopathic doctor on the Rez [reservation]. Now I
hope in the future to encourage new nurses and doctors to accept some
of our major needs. This includes not cutting my hair if I don't want to

have it cut or shaved. They should make sure to include me in things that are happening and to have conversations with me. Don't just talk – listen. Build a relationship with me and then we can work together. Also it would be very important to us if there was a spare room, it could be called a spiritual room. Just like the *sema7* [white people] have a chapel at the hospital,[1] we would like a room like that where we could have our privacy, play our drums, sing our spiritual songs, smudge, and do our spiritual thing like the sema7 does his. This way we could have eight or ten people visiting without disturbing others. My first major acceptance of my various illnesses in life is when I went to my first sweat. I started to heal big time and I shed many a tear while sweating or while in the sweat. So we should encourage all Elders to participate in sweats – this includes Elders with memory loss or dementia. Maybe a nurse could take an Elder to a sweat. Or a senior citizens' home could build a sweat out back. If this happens, then we can thank the Creator for caring people.

And the language. Even though I can't speak my language fluent, I can speak a few words. And I would like to see all of us speaking our language. They could train a few of the Native nurses to speak our language – that would help us feel respected. Encourage us, spend time with us – visit us more often. Show us that you care and that you understand where we're coming from, that being hurt in the past carries forward into the future. Look at the damage that was caused and the toll that was taken on my parents. This carries on and on, and the hurt has to stop. And if the emotional bruises are healed – through sweats, smudging, love, and the Creator – then the dementia can be healed or the impact of living with it lessened. All things in the body can be healed, and with perseverance and determination a person with dementia can slow down or heal most of the effects of it and lead a healthy life. I heard the sema7 call this "rementia."[2] We call it healing.

Notes

1   Depending on the dialect, which varies by location in Secwepemc territory, sema7 may be spelled *shéma* in Secwepemcstín. For example, an Elder from the south spelled it this way during earlier research (see Hulko et al. 2010).
2   See Sixsmith, Stilwell, and Copeland (1993).

References

Hulko, W., E. Camille, E. Antifeau, M. Arnouse, N. Bachynksi, and D. Taylor. 2010. "Views of First Nation Elders on Memory Loss and Memory Care in Later Life." *Journal of Cross-Cultural Gerontology* 25 (4): 317–42. DOI:10.1007/s10823-010-9123-9.

Sixsmith, A., J. Stilwell, and J. Copeland. 1993. "'Rementia': Challenging the Limits of Dementia Care." *International Journal of Geriatric Psychiatry* 8 (12): 993–1000.

PART 1

PREVALENCE, CAUSES, AND PUBLIC DISCOURSE

CHAPTER 1

CURRENT AND PROJECTED DEMENTIA PREVALENCE

in First Nations Populations in Canada

Jennifer Walker and Kristen Jacklin

DEMENTIA IS EMERGING as a significant health concern globally and in Canada.[1] Approximately half a million Canadians have dementia, and it has been estimated that their numbers will more than double over the next thirty years (Alzheimer Society of Canada 2010). Data on dementia in Indigenous populations are scarce, but Indigenous health organizations in Ontario began noting rising rates in 2007, as well as the need for more data to help them ensure that health and social planning supported Indigenous communities, families, and individuals (Sutherland 2007).[2] Responding to this call and to a request from Health Canada's First Nations and Inuit Home and Community Care program, we offer an overview of published information on the epidemiology of dementia in Canadian First Nations. We also outline an approach, using available data, for estimating current rates and projecting future trends that could be applied to other communities and nations.

Prevalence

Although dementia is expected to be an increasing challenge for First Nations in Canada, few published reports have discussed its epidemiology in these populations. Early work in North America suggested that Alzheimer's disease (AD) may be less prevalent in Indigenous communities than in non-

Indigenous ones, partially owing to genetic influences (Henderson et al. 2002; Hendrie et al. 1993), and that vascular dementia may be more common than other forms due to high rates of vascular risk factors (Hendrie et al. 1993). In one Canadian study, Hugh Hendrie et al. (1993) surveyed and assessed 192 Cree seniors from Norway House and Nelson House in northern Manitoba. They found that the age-standardized prevalence of AD was lower for the Cree participants (0.5 percent) than for Manitoba seniors who were not Indigenous (3.5 percent). However, age-standardized prevalence for all dementia was 4.2 percent for both populations. Thus, the early work indicated that dementia was as common among First Nations as it was in other Canadian populations and that vascular dementia, not AD, was the primary driver for the rates among Indigenous people.

More recent estimates, grounded in administrative health care data in Alberta and British Columbia (British Columbia Provincial Health Officer 2009; Jacklin, Walker, and Shawande 2013), provide information on the prevalence of treated dementia, based on a recorded physician diagnosis. These analyses indicate that the age-standardized prevalence of dementia among First Nations people who are registered under the Indian Act is increasing more quickly than in the non–First Nations population (Figure 1.1). In fact, dementia among First Nations appears to have increased to meet the level of the non–First Nations population (British Columbia Provincial Health Officer 2009), or even to have surpassed it by an estimated 34 percent (Jacklin, Walker, and Shawande 2013). Whereas, in general, aging is the most important risk factor for dementia, the results suggest that First Nations patients develop dementia at a younger age than their non–First Nations counterparts (British Columbia Provincial Health Officer 2009; Jacklin, Walker, and Shawande 2013). Figure 1.2 illustrates this relationship, based on 2,074 First Nations people and 175,518 non–First Nations individuals in Alberta who were diagnosed with dementia between 1998 and 2009. Additionally, in the general population, women are more likely than men to develop dementia, whereas the diagnosis rate for First Nations men is higher than for the general population (Figure 1.1) (British Columbia Provincial Health Officer 2009; Jacklin, Walker, and Shawande 2013).

Expected Trends

These emerging patterns in Canada, coupled with demographic projections, will probably result in a further upsurge in dementia and an accompanying need for increased culturally appropriate care. The most recent population

FIGURE 1.1 Age-standardized prevalence of physician-treated dementia among First Nations and non–First Nations people, Alberta, 1998–2009

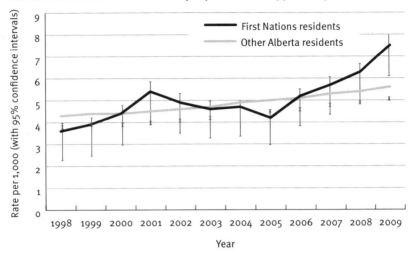

Source: Adapted from Jacklin, Walker, and Shawande (2013), with permission of the Canadian Public Health Association. Data from Alberta Health Physician Claims Data and Alberta Health Care Insurance Plan Population Registry, Primary diagnosis of dementia (ICD-9 code 290 or 331.0).

FIGURE 1.2 Age-specific prevalence of physician-treated dementia among First Nations and non–First Nations people, Alberta, 1998–2009 combined

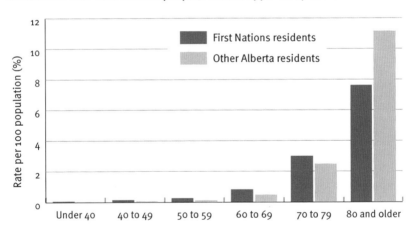

Source: Jacklin, Walker, and Shawande (2013), reproduced with permission of the Canadian Public Health Association. Data from Alberta Health Physician Claims Data and Alberta Health Care Insurance Plan Population Registry, Primary diagnosis of dementia (ICD-9 code 290 or 331.0).

projections show that the number of First Nations people in Canada is expected to rise by 1.4 times between 2006 and 2031 (Caron Malenfant and Morency 2011). A disproportionate amount of this growth will be among those aged sixty and older, whose numbers are expected to increase by 3.4 times, from 54,165 in 2006 to 184,334 in 2031 (Caron Malenfant and Morency 2011). This shifting age structure will probably have a large impact on the prevalence of dementia in First Nations populations.

Further exacerbation of this trend may arise from the higher than average incidence of other dementia risk factors among First Nations people. There is no single cause of dementia. Although genetic factors play an important role, only 5–7 percent of AD patients have a clear diagnosis of the genetic familial type of the disease (Alzheimer Society of Canada 2010). In rare situations, some First Nations in Canada exhibit specific familial AD (Butler et al. 2011). More commonly, dementia occurs due to a combination of genetic and environmental risk factors that exist throughout the lifespan (Arkles et al. 2010; Diamond 2008; Patterson et al. 2007). In general, First Nations people experience a confluence of factors throughout their lives that have been associated with dementia. Among these are low vaccination rates (Martens et al. 2002), low formal educational attainment (St. Germain and Dyck 2011), high rates of head injury (First Nations Information Governance Centre 2011), and exposure to poverty and psychosocial stressors (First Nations Information Governance Centre 2011; Reading 2009), including post-traumatic stress disorder related to residential schools (Brave Heart 2003; Brave Heart and DeBruyn 1998; Hulko et al. 2010).

Additionally, First Nations populations have high rates of chronic conditions, such as hypertension, obesity, and diabetes (First Nations Information Governance Centre 2011). Recent evidence indicates that people with type 2 diabetes have up to nearly two times higher risk of developing dementia later in life than people without type 2 diabetes (Ohara et al. 2011). Population-based researchers have observed that the age-adjusted prevalence rate for type 2 diabetes among First Nations is approximately four times higher than for the general population (Dyck et al. 2010; Green et al. 2003). In some age and sex groups, this ratio is up to seven times higher (Green et al. 2003). Even with hypothetical interventions that would decrease the incidence of type 2 diabetes over the next several decades, it is still expected to expand at a faster rate among First Nations as the population growth outpaces mortality in the middle and late age groups (Green et al. 2003). At a population level, First Nations people also experience higher risk of chronic-disease-associated lifestyle factors, such as smoking, drug misuse, alcohol-related disorders, and low levels of physical activity, that have been associated with dementia (First Nations Information Governance Centre 2011; Reading 2009). Many of these are related to poverty, community-level risk factors, and the effects of intergenerational trauma (Reading and Wein 2013).

Closing the Information Gap

Our initial review for Health Canada revealed a number of limitations in estimating the prevalence of dementia in the First Nations population. Among these were poor and limited health information systems for Aboriginal people in Canada (Minore, Katt, and Hill 2009). In addition, questions concerning dementia and neurological health were not included in the national health surveys that were administered to Aboriginal people (Jacklin and Walker 2012). In reviewing the various health surveys that are routinely employed for First Nations groups, we found that questions concerning a dementia diagnosis or even a variable on memory did not exist for on-reserve groups (e.g., Regional Health Survey) or did not sample sufficient numbers of off-reserve First Nations populations to allow reporting of dementia (e.g., Canadian Community Health Survey). Also, in the majority of provinces, administrative health data often lack the elements that are necessary to identify First Nations, Inuit, or Métis patients. In a few cases, First Nations people who are registered status Indians have been identified within provincial insurance and billing systems, using unique identifiers in four Canadian provinces (Alberta, British Columbia, Saskatchewan, and Manitoba). However, other provinces' and territories' analyses of First Nations administrative data is limited to specific projects and is often costly and complex (Minore, Katt, and Hill 2009). In all cases, the analysis of First Nations–identified administrative data should be subject to the principles of OCAP® (ownership, control, access, and possession) (First Nations Information Governance Centre 2018). OCAP® principles were developed by First Nations organizations in 1998 in recognition of the collective rights of First Nations to govern the use of information about themselves. The application of OCAP® can ensure that the analysis and interpretation of health data are conducted within an understanding of colonization. This helps to ensure that data on dementia rates are viewed in the context of social and economic structures, not simply within an individualized framework of risk behaviour.

Currently, the available data concerning the prevalence of dementia in

First Nations populations are from administrative health datasets in Alberta and British Columbia. These rely on a physician diagnosis of dementia, which has limitations in measuring prevalence among First Nations. For non-Indigenous populations, physician-diagnosed dementia has been routinely used in health services research and reporting (Ho et al. 2011). In general, the diagnosis is largely "a clinical exercise"; that is, the condition cannot be detected via a simple test (Robillard 2007; Third Canadian Consensus Conference 2007). Because there is no accepted definitive test for AD (except autopsy after death), reaching a diagnosis involves an integrative approach (various assessments). It usually entails the exclusion of all other probable causes by laboratory and/or imaging tests. Typically, patients presenting with dementia are evaluated during a clinical visit with a physician. Physicians evaluate these patients based on the symptoms reported by them or their family members, their functioning, and any changes over time (Weiner and Lipton 2012). According to the Third Canadian Consensus Conference on Diagnosis and Treatment of Dementia (2007), the recommended examination for dementia includes the following (Robillard 2007; Weiner and Lipton 2012):

- history taking and physical exam (including neurological examination – olfactory, visual, auditory, facial muscles, motor system, parkinsonism, sensation, reflexes, gait, and posture)
- mental state exam
- laboratory work (blood and urine)
- and, only if indicated (i.e., selective use of)
  ‣ structural neuroimaging: CT and MRI
  ‣ functional neuroimaging: PET or SPECT scanning.

Because the availability and accessibility of these health services vary for First Nations across Canada, physician diagnosis is not necessarily a good basis for estimating prevalence. Rural and remote First Nations may have infrequent access to physician examinations, and doctors in these locales are rarely trained in geriatric medicine (Morgan et al. 2009). Though First Nations people residing off-reserve may have easier access to physicians, they can experience many enduring barriers, rooted in systemic racism (Health Council of Canada 2012). They report visiting a physician significantly less often than non-Indigenous people (Garner et al. 2010). In all health care settings, even if access to specialized geriatric care is available, systemic barriers related to Indigenous status nonetheless remain (Buchignani and Armstrong-Esther 1999). Health care systems are generally culturally incongruent with the needs of First Nations people (Cammer 2006; Chapleski, Sobeck, and Fisher 2003; Jervis and Manson 2002), which contributes to a lack of culturally safe dementia care for them. With these factors in mind, one would expect physician diagnosis to underestimate the prevalence of dementia, particularly for First Nations people.

Despite these limitations, administrative data reflect a total population approach to estimating the absolute and relative numbers of First Nations and non–First Nations people who have been diagnosed with and treated for dementia. The analysis that we describe and present in this chapter is an initial estimate and projection for the prevalence of physician-treated dementia among the First Nations of Canada, based on available information. We developed a simple model to quantify the expected impact of population aging on the prevalence and crude number of First Nations people with dementia over a twenty-five-year period.

Approaches to Understanding the Impact of Dementia

We used prevalence data for physician-treated dementia from one province (Alberta) to estimate the number of First Nations people who were being treated for the condition in all of Canada (Jacklin, Walker, and Shawande 2013). We also used national First Nations population projection data published by Statistics Canada to approximate the impact of population aging on the prevalence estimates (Caron Malenfant and Morency 2011). As an additional source of information, we incorporated projections published by the Alzheimer Society of Canada (2010) that examined the potential impact of population-level interventions to change the long-term outcomes for the expected increase in dementia.

Estimating Current Dementia Prevalence

We used the most recent published estimates of physician-treated dementia for First Nations, which are based on administrative data from the Surveillance and Assessment Branch of Alberta Health and Wellness (Jacklin, Walker, and Shawande 2013). The data were collaboratively analyzed and interpreted by a trained First Nations epidemiologist, in consultation with the National Aboriginal Health Organization and under the guidance of an Elder. For First Nations people in Alberta, the age-specific prevalence rates of treated dementia were as follows: 0.8 percent for ages sixty to sixty-nine, 3.0 percent for ages seventy to seventy-nine, and 7.6 percent for age eighty and older (Jacklin, Walker, and Shawande 2013).

Estimating the Projected Dementia Prevalence

The second key data source was the population projections from Statistics Canada for First Nations, Inuit, and Métis (Caron Malenfant and Morency 2011), which were based on the 2006 census and projected out to 2031. In making these projections, Statistics Canada assumed that no ethnic migration would occur, that fertility rates would remain constant, and that internal migration rates would not differ appreciably from those of the past decade. For more details on Statistics Canada's projection methodology, please see Éric Caron Malenfant and Jean-Dominique Morency (2011). To obtain comparative projections for the general Canadian population, we combined information from other Statistics Canada reports, assuming a medium growth scenario (that fertility and immigration rates would resemble those of recent years and that life expectancy would moderately increase) (Statistics Canada 2010; Statistics Canada – CANSIM 2010).

For the purposes of the numeric projection results, we worked from the conservative assumption that the age-specific prevalence of dementia among First Nations and Inuit would not change between 2006 and 2031. Thus, the projected numbers primarily reflect the impact of population aging, which remains the most important driver of dementia rates, and do *not* account for any increase in age-specific prevalence that may arise from increased risk factor exposure, such as diabetes. We also assumed that neither the likelihood of recognition and diagnosis of dementia nor the accuracy of diagnostic coding for dementia by hospitals and physicians would change over time.

Estimating the Impact of Population-Based Prevention Efforts

The third source of information was the Alzheimer Society of Canada's "Rising Tide" (2010) report, which outlines the potential effects of two prevention-intervention scenarios on nation-wide rates of dementia over time. The report projected that if Canadians aged sixty-five and older who did not have dementia but who were already moderately to highly active increased their physical activity levels by 50 percent, dementia would decrease by 5.1 percent over ten years and by 8.6 percent over thirty years. It also estimated that a delay of two years in the onset of dementia would result in 21.6 percent fewer Canadians with dementia over ten years and 36.4 percent fewer over thirty years (Alzheimer Society of Canada 2010).

Current and Expected Trends in Dementia in First Nations Populations

Extrapolating from the published dementia rates for First Nations people in Alberta, we estimate that in 2006, approximately 1,179 First Nations people in Canada were being treated for dementia. About 539 of them were living on-reserve (Table 1.1).

The previously discussed population aging trends will contribute to a 4.0 times increase from 1,179 to 4,723 in the number of First Nations people being treated for dementia (Table 1.1). This tendency will be highest on-reserve, where numbers are expected to rise from 539 to 2,474, a 4.6-fold increase. With a 50 percent increase in physical activity levels among First Nations seniors without dementia who are already moderately to highly active, the projected number of people living with dementia in 2031 would drop by 583. This would represent a twenty-five-year increase of 3.5 times (from 1,179 to 4,140), instead of 4.0 times.

TABLE 1.1 Estimated prevalence of treated dementia in First Nations, 2006 and 2031

	Estimated treated dementia (#)		Projected increase: 2006 to 2031
	2006	2031	
60–69 years	261	760	2.9 times
70–79 years	476	1,855	3.9 times
80 years and older	442	2,108	4.8 times
Total aged 60 and older	1,179	4,723	4.0 times
On-reserve aged 60 and older	539	2,474	4.6 times

If the onset of dementia were delayed by two years, the projected number of First Nations seniors aged sixty and older living with dementia in 2031 would be reduced by 2,467. Thus, the projected increase would be a mere doubling, from 1,179 to 2,256 over twenty-five years.

Basing our conclusions on the rates of physician-treated dementia in Alberta and population projections for First Nations, we estimate that population aging alone will result in a 4.0-fold increase in the number of First Nations people aged sixty and older who are being treated for dementia by 2031. This is in comparison to the 2.3-fold increase that is expected for the general Canadian population. Future refinements to this model would require incorporation of the impact of the changing profile of dementia risk factors in First Nations, such as type 2 diabetes, rising levels of educational attainment, and geographical migration to urban centres.

These estimates are based on administrative health data, which rely on the accurate diagnosis and coding of dementia. Research on the diagnosis of dementia for Indigenous people in North America suggests that under-diagnosis may be a considerable issue (Hendrie 2006; Jervis and Manson 2002, 2007; Morgan et al. 2009). For example, screening for AD is often not viewed as a priority for physicians (Powell 2002). Similarly, a diagnosis may not always be a priority or be valued by an Indigenous person, who may hold differing views from the physician on the meaning of the illness or for whom other social inequalities may take precedence (Pollitt 1997). A US study shows that, on average, American Indians experience symptoms for five years before they seek a diagnosis, whereas Euro-Americans consult a doctor after two years (Dilworth-Anderson 2010). Late and under-diagnosis of dementia is believed to be related to the "naturalized" explanatory model of illness that some Indigenous peoples hold, where the early stages of dementia are not viewed as a disease or health issue (Griffin-Pierce et al. 2008). It may also arise due to the avoidance of health care systems because of mistrust and poor past relations between physicians and Indigenous people (Griffin-Pierce et al. 2008). Poor access to diagnostic services plays a role as well (Morgan et al. 2009; Weiner, Rossetti, and Harrah 2011).

Further, an important component of the diagnostic process is the mental state exam used for screening. Certain screening tests are more relevant cross-culturally than others (Borson et al. 1999), and the inappropriateness of cross-cultural screening instruments is a long-recognized problem. Issues include the following: fairness of tests that are translated into other languages (for example, words can be more or less complex in other languages); relevance of the items on a test (such as the name of the prime minister or familiarity with animal symbols); educational history; and cross-cultural meanings of test items (Cattarinich, Gibson, and Cave 2001; Griffin-Pierce et al. 2008; Kaufert and Shapiro 1996). Cross-cultural research studies show that the Mini-Mental State Examination, one of the most widely used screening tests, is more affected by culture, language, and education level than other screening tests (Borson et al. 1999, 2005). To improve accuracy, assessing dementia and its associated risk factors must take into account an

Indigenous determinants of health perspective across the life course. Such a framework recognizes a holistic view of health in the context of First Nations communities and their complex historic and contemporary social realities (Reading and Wein 2013). To this end, there are alternative screening tools, some of which have been developed by or with Indigenous people (Hulko et al. 2010; Lanting et al. 2011). However, their use is not widespread and would not yet affect the validity of the diagnosis data in the administrative dataset.

Despite limitations to the data that these screening and diagnostic practices produce, the results point to an estimated fourfold increase in dementia-related service needs for First Nations seniors. Presently, First Nations communities have few resources to provide appropriate care for people with dementia (Sutherland 2007). Dementia care is complex and requires several co-ordinated services: home support (meals, housework), personal support, nursing support, day programs, specialist referrals and monitoring, medication, safety monitoring, and respite. In the case of First Nations seniors, dementia care also involves Indigenous traditional healing practices. Also, dementia is often co-morbid with one or more other chronic conditions, such as type 2 diabetes, heart disease, arthritis, and cerebrovascular disease, which further elevates care needs. This increasing requirement for dementia care has implications for health care policy and planning, community-based programming, and culturally safe dementia screening, diagnosis, and care (Jacklin and Walker 2012).

The projections may also be used to inform policy and program development aimed at preventing dementia in First Nations populations. Importantly, our application of the Alzheimer Society of Canada's (2010) intervention findings suggests that, theoretically, increasing physical activity and measures to delay the onset of dementia could dramatically change the progression of the condition in First Nations. Of course, any similar interventions in First Nations would need to be appropriate to the community, culture, and context (see also Chapter 4, this volume). Among the key prevention measures for dementia is maintaining cardiovascular health through regular exercise (Ahlskog et al. 2011; Barak and Aizenberg 2010; Hughes and Ganguli 2009; Larson et al. 2006) and the management of hypertension via pharmacologic and other approaches (Barak and Aizenberg 2010; Cooper 2002). Cognitive engagement also appears to prevent or delay dementia (Barak and Aizenberg 2010; Hughes and Ganguli 2009). Other promising prevention measures include healthy eating, moderation in alcohol use, and abstinence from smoking (Hughes and Ganguli 2009). Likewise, interventions to reduce the incidence of type 2 diabetes and to better manage pre-diabetes could mitigate some of the projected increase in dementia in First Nations. Effective community-based approaches to population health improvements, such as the Kahnawake Schools Diabetes Prevention Project (Salsberg et al. 2008), can have enduring and wide-reaching success in First Nations.

❖❖❖

The analyses presented here underscore the challenge of using limited data to answer complex questions. At present, communities and service providers lack the necessary information for an effective response to the rising levels of dementia among First Nations in Canada. This chapter emphasizes the need for more accurate diagnosis, better understandings of risk associations, and improved collection and use of dementia-related information. Despite the shortcomings of the data and the probable underestimation of the prevalence of dementia, the current state of knowledge is that dementia rates are rising among First Nations, that the age- and sex-related patterns for First Nations differ from those for non-Indigenous groups, and that the projected increases for First Nations are roughly double those for the general population.

This evidence may be used as a platform in developing a First Nations–driven comprehensive plan for the collection of data to assess dementia risk, prevalence, and outcomes as well as community- or system-level responses to expected dementia increases. If deemed a priority by First Nations, any work in this area must adhere to the OCAP® principles and be driven by the experiences, needs, and expectations of First Nations people and communities. This complex undertaking involves many partners and jurisdictions, and is best led by (or in close partnership with) First Nations organizations, which have the depth and breadth of understanding to best employ OCAP®. A national surveillance program would require strategic collaboration between many groups, including First Nations leadership and organizations, geriatricians, federal and provincial governments, researchers, community-based workers, and families and individuals dealing with dementia, among others. However, small and meaningful steps can be taken toward this larger goal of better dementia diagnosis and improved collection and use of data by everyone involved in providing or planning care for older First Nations people.

Notes

1   The term "dementia" refers to irreversible and progressive conditions: Alzheimer's disease (AD), vascular dementia, mixed dementia, Lewy body dementia, frontotemporal dementia, Wernicke-Korsakoff syndrome, and Creutzfeldt-Jakob disease (Alzheimer Society of Canada 2010; Weiner and Lipton 2012).

2   In this chapter, "Indigenous" refers to people whose ancestors originally inhabited the territory that is now Canada. It encompasses First Nations, Inuit, and Métis populations.

References

Ahlskog, J.E., Y.E. Geda, N.R. Graff-Radford, and R.C. Petersen. 2011. "Physical Exercise as a Preventive or Disease-Modifying Treatment of Dementia and Brain Aging." *Mayo Clinic Proceedings* 86 (9): 876–84.

Alzheimer Society of Canada. 2010. "Rising Tide: The Impact of Dementia on Canadian Society." http://alzheimer.ca/sites/default/files/files/chapters-on/york/rising_tide_full_report_eng_final.pdf.

Arkles, Rachelle, Lisa Jackson Pulver, Hamish Robertson, Brian Draper, Simon Chalkley, and G.A. (Tony) Broe. 2010. "Ageing, Cognition and Dementia in Australian Aboriginal and Torres Strait Islander Peoples: A Life Cycle Approach." http://www.dementiaresearch.org.au/images/dcrc/output-files/260-ipwd1_monograph.pdf.

Barak, Yoram, and Dov Aizenberg. 2010. "Is Dementia Preventable? Focus on Alzheimer's Disease." *Expert Review of Neurotherapeutics* 10 (11): 1689–98.

Borson, S., M. Brush, E. Gil, J. Scanlan, P. Vitaliano, J. Chen, J. Cashman, M.M. Sta Maria, R. Barnhart, and J. Roques. 1999. "The Clock Drawing Test: Utility for Dementia Detection in Multiethnic Elders." *Journals of Gerontology Series A: Biomedical Sciences and Medical Sciences* 54 (11): M534–40.

Borson, S., J.M. Scanlan, J. Watanabe, S.P. Tu, and M. Lessig. 2005. "Simplifying Detection of Cognitive Impairment: Comparison of the Mini-Cog and Mini-Mental State Examination in a Multiethnic Sample." *Journal of the American Geriatrics Society* 53 (5): 871–74.

Brave Heart, M. Yellow Horse. 2003. "The Historical Trauma Response among Natives and Its Relationship with Substance Abuse: A Lakota Illustration." *Journal of Psychoactive Drugs* 35 (1): 7–13.

Brave Heart, M. Yellow Horse, and L.M. DeBruyn. 1998. "The American Indian Holocaust: Healing Historical Unresolved Grief." *American Indian and Alaska Native Mental Health Research* 8 (2): 60–82.

British Columbia Provincial Health Officer. 2009. *Pathways to Healing – 2nd Report on the Health and Well-Being of Aboriginal People in British Columbia. Provincial Health Officer's Annual Report 2007.* Victoria: Ministry of Healthy Living and Sport. http://www.health.gov.bc.ca/pho/pdf/abohlth11-var7.pdf.

Buchignani, Norman, and Christopher Armstrong-Esther. 1999. "Informal Care and Older Native Canadians." *Ageing and Society* 19 (1): 3–32.

Butler, Rachel, Emily Dwosh, B. Lynn Beattie, Colleen Guimond, Sofia Lombera,

Elana Brief, Judy Illes, and A. Dessa Sadovnick. 2011. "Genetic Counseling for Early-Onset Familial Alzheimer Disease in Large Aboriginal Kindred from a Remote Community in British Columbia: Unique Challenges and Possible Solutions." *Journal of Genetic Counseling* 20 (2): 136–42.

Cammer, Allison Lee. 2006. "Negotiating Culturally Incongruent Healthcare Systems: The Process of Accessing Dementia Care in Northern Saskatchewan." Master's thesis, University of Saskatchewan. http://hdl.handle.net/10388/etd-12192006-160831.

Caron Malenfant, Éric, and Jean-Dominique Morency. 2011. *Population Projections by Aboriginal Identity in Canada, 2006 to 2031.* Ottawa: Statistics Canada.

Cattarinich, X., N. Gibson, and A.J. Cave. 2001. "Assessing Mental Capacity in Canadian Aboriginal Seniors." *Social Science and Medicine* 53 (11): 1469–79.

Chapleski, E.E., J. Sobeck, and C. Fisher. 2003. "Long-Term Care Preferences and Attitudes among Great Lakes American Indian Families: Cultural Context Matters." *Care Management Journals* 4 (2): 94–100.

Cooper, B. 2002. "Thinking Preventively about Dementia: A Review." *International Journal of Geriatric Psychiatry* 17 (10): 895–906.

Diamond, Jack. 2008. *A Report on Alzheimer's Disease and Current Research.* Toronto: Alzheimer Society of Canada.

Dilworth-Anderson, Peggye. 2010. "Diagnosis of Alzheimer's within Cultural Context." *Alzheimer's and Dementia* 6 (4): S95.

Dyck, Roland, Nathaniel Osgood, Ting Hsiang Lin, Amy Gao, and Mary Rose Stang. 2010. "Epidemiology of Diabetes Mellitus among First Nations and Non-First Nations Adults." *Canadian Medical Association Journal* 183 (3): 249–55.

First Nations Information Governance Centre. 2011. *RHS Phase 2 (2008/10) Preliminary Results.* Ottawa: First Nations Information Governance Centre. http://fnigc.ca/sites/default/files/RHSPreliminaryReport.pdf.

–. 2018. *The First Nations Principles of OCAP®.* Ottawa: First Nations Information Governance Centre. https://fnigc.ca/ocapr.html.

Garner, Rochelle, Gisèle Carrière, Claudia Sanmartin, and Longitudinal Health and Administrative Data Research Team. 2010. *The Health of Inuit, Métis and First Nations Adults Living Off-Reserve in Canada: The Impact of Socio-economic Status on Inequalities in Health.* Health Research Working Paper Series, Catalogue No. 82-622-X No. 004. Ottawa: Statistics Canada.

Green, Chris, James F. Blanchard, T. Kue Young, and Jane Griffith. 2003. "The Epidemiology of Diabetes in the Manitoba-Registered First Nation Population." *Diabetes Care* 26 (7): 1993–98.

Griffin-Pierce, Trudy, Nina Silverberg, Donald Connor, Minnie Jim, Jill Peters, Alfred Kaszniak, and Marwan N. Sabbagh. 2008. "Challenges to the Recognition and Assessment of Alzheimer's Disease in American Indians of the Southwestern United States." *Alzheimer's and Dementia* 4 (4): 291–99.

Health Council of Canada. 2012. *Empathy, Dignity, and Respect: Creating Cultural Safety for Aboriginal People in Urban Health Care.* Toronto: Health Council of Canada.

Henderson, J. Neil, Richard Crook, Julia Crook, John Hardy, Luisa Onstead, Linda

Carson-Henderson, Pat Mayer, Bea Parker, Ronald Petersen, and Birdie Williams. 2002. "Apolipoprotein E4 and Tau Allele Frequencies among Choctaw Indians." *Neuroscience Letters* 324 (1): 77–79.

Hendrie, Hugh C. 2006. "Lessons Learned from International Comparative Crosscultural Studies on Dementia." *American Journal of Geriatric Psychiatry* 14 (6): 480–88. DOI:10.1097/01.JGP.0000192497.81296.fb.

Hendrie, Hugh C., et al. 1993. "Alzheimer's Disease Is Rare in Cree." *International Psychogeriatrics* 5 (1): 5–14.

Ho, M.M., X. Camacho, A. Gruneir, and S.E. Bronskill. 2011. "Overview of Cohorts: Definitions and Study Methodology." In *Health System Use by Frail Ontario Seniors: An In-Depth Examination of Four Vulnerable Cohorts,* ed. S.E. Bronskill, X. Camacho, A. Gruneir, and M.M. Ho, 6–28. Toronto: Institute for Clinical Evaluative Sciences.

Hughes, Tiffany F., and Mary Ganguli. 2009. "Modifiable Midlife Risk Factors for Late-Life Cognitive Impairment and Dementia." *Current Psychiatry Review* 5 (2): 73–92.

Hulko, Wendy, Evelyn Camille, Elisabeth Antifeau, Mike Arnouse, Nicole Bachynksi, and Denise Taylor. 2010. "Views of First Nation Elders on Memory Loss and Memory Care in Later Life." *Journal of Cross-Cultural Gerontology* 25 (4): 317–42. DOI:10.1007/s10823-010-9123-9.

Jacklin, Kristen, and Jennifer Walker. 2012. "Trends in Alzheimer's Disease and Related Dementias among First Nations and Inuit: Final Report." Report submitted to First Nations and Inuit Home and Community Care Program, Health Canada.

Jacklin, Kristen M., Jennifer D. Walker, and Marjory Shawande. 2013. "The Emergence of Dementia as a Health Concern among First Nations Populations in Alberta, Canada." *Canadian Journal of Public Health* 104 (1): e39–e44.

Jervis, Lori L., and Spero M. Manson. 2002. "American Indians/Alaska Natives and Dementia." *Alzheimer Disease and Associated Disorders* 16 (2): S89–S95.

–. 2007. "Cognitive Impairment, Psychiatric Disorders, and Problematic Behaviors in a Tribal Nursing Home." *Journal of Aging and Health* 19 (2): 260–74.

Kaufert, Joseph M., and Evelyn Shapiro. 1996. "Cultural, Linguistic and Contextual Factors in Validating the Mental Status Questionnaire: The Experience of Aboriginal Elders in Manitoba." *Transcultural Psychiatry* 33 (3): 277–96.

Lanting, Shawnda, Margaret Crossley, Debra Morgan, and Allison Cammer. 2011. "Aboriginal Experiences of Aging and Dementia in a Context of Sociocultural Change: Qualitative Analysis of Key Informant Group Interviews with Aboriginal Seniors." *Journal of Cross-Cultural Gerontology* 26 (1): 103–17.

Larson, Eric B., Li Wang, James D. Bowen, Wayne C. McCormick, Linda Teri, Paul Crane, and Walter Kukull. 2006. "Exercise Is Associated with Reduced Risk for Incident Dementia among Persons 65 Years of Age and Older." *Annals of Internal Medicine* 144 (2): 73–81.

Martens, Patricia, et al. 2002. *The Health and Health Care Use of Registered First Nations People Living in Manitoba: A Population-Based Study.* Manitoba Centre for Health Policy, University of Manitoba. http://mchp-appserv.cpe.umanitoba.ca/reference/rfn_report.pdf.

Minore, B., M. Katt, and M.E. Hill. 2009. "Planning without Facts: Ontario's Aboriginal Health Information Challenge." *Journal of Agromedicine* 14 (2): 90–96.

Morgan, Debra G., et al. 2009. "Improving Access to Dementia Care: Development and Evaluation of a Rural and Remote Memory Clinic." *Aging and Mental Health* 13 (1): 17–30.

Ohara, T., Y. Doi, T. Ninomiya, Y. Hirakawa, J. Hata, T. Iwaki, S. Kanba, and Y. Kiyohara. 2011. "Glucose Tolerance Status and Risk of Dementia in the Community: The Hisayama Study." *Neurology* 77: 1126–34.

Patterson, Christopher , John Feightner, Angeles Garcia, and Chris MacKnight. 2007. "General Risk Factors for Dementia: A Systematic Evidence Review." *Alzheimer's and Dementia* 3 (4): 341–47. DOI:10.1016/j.jalz.2007.07.001.

Pollitt, P.A. 1997. "The Problem of Dementia in Australian Aboriginal and Torres Strait Islander Communities: An Overview." *International Journal of Geriatric Psychiatry* 12 (2): 155–63.

Powell, Artuss L. 2002. "On Issues Pertinent to Alzheimer Disease and Cultural Diversity." *Alzheimer Disease and Associated Disorders* 16 (suppl. 2): S43–S45.

Reading, Charlotte Loppie, and Fred Wein. 2013. *Health Inequalities and Social Determinants of Aboriginal Peoples' Health.* Prince George, BC: National Collaborating Centre for Aboriginal Health. First published 2009. https://www.ccnsa-nccah.ca/docs/determinants/RPT-HealthInequalities-Reading-Wien-EN.pdf.

Reading, J. 2009. *The Crisis of Chronic Disease among Aboriginal Peoples: A Challenge for Public Health, Population Health and Social Policy.* Centre for Aboriginal Health Research, University of Victoria. https://dspace.library.uvic.ca/bitstream/handle/1828/5380/Chronic-Disease-2009.pdf.

Robillard, Alain. 2007. "Clinical Diagnosis of Dementia." *Alzheimer's and Dementia* 3 (4): 292–98. DOI:10.1016/j.jalz.2007.08.002.

Salsberg, Jon, Stanley Louttit, Alex M. McComber, Roderick Fiddler, Mariam Naqshbandi, Olivier Receveur, Stewart B. Harris, and Ann C. Macaulay. 2008. "Knowledge, Capacity and Readiness: Translating Successful Experiences in Community-Based Participatory Research for Health Promotion." *Pimatisiwin: A Journal of Indigenous and Aboriginal Community Health* 5 (2): 125–50.

St. Germain, Gerry, and Lillian Eva Dyck. 2011. "Reforming First Nations Education: From Crisis to Hope." Report of the Standing Senate Committee on Aboriginal Peoples. http://www.parl.gc.ca/Content/SEN/Committee/411/appa/rep/rep03dec11-e.pdf.

Statistics Canada. 2010. "Profile of Census Divisions/Census Subdivisions." 2006 Census of Population, Catalogue No. 94-575-XCB2006001. Statistics Canada.

Statistics Canada – CANSIM. 2010. "Projected Population by Age Group and Sex According to Three Projection Scenarios for 2010, 2011, 2016, 2021, 2026, 2031 and 2036, at July 1." Table 052-0005 and Catalogue No. 91-520-X. Statistics Canada.

Sutherland, M.E. 2007, March. "Alzheimer's Disease and Related Dementias (ADRD) in Aboriginal Communities: New Visions and Understandings." Paper presented at Alzheimer's Disease and Related Dementias within Aboriginal Individuals – Roundtable Forum, Sudbury, ON.

Third Canadian Consensus Conference on Diagnosis and Treatment of Dementia Steering Committee. 2007. "146 Approved Recommendations Final – July, 2007." http://www.cccdtd.ca/pdfs/final_recommendations_cccdtd_2007.pdf.

Weiner, Myron F., and Anne M. Lipton. 2012. *Clinical Manual of Alzheimer's Disease and Other Dementias.* Arlington: American Psychiatric Association.

Weiner, Myron F., Heidi C. Rossetti, and Kasia Harrah. 2011. "Videoconference Diagnosis and Management of Choctaw Indian Dementia Patients." *Alzheimer's and Dementia* 7 (6): 562–66.

CHAPTER 2

INDIGENOUS VASCULAR DEMENTIA
An Indigenous Syndemic Dementia Model

J. Neil Henderson, Linda D. Carson, and Kama King

INDIGENOUS PEOPLE IN NORTH AMERICA have only recently been the subject of late-life cognitive impairment research, which has tended to have three focal points: the general population of Canada and the United Sates, cross-cultural perspectives (international and domestic), and Indigenous perspectives from North America. The analytic models employed by most of this research are based on the premise that disease is a cultural construction. These analyses do not necessarily exclude biological factors, but they do emphasize social and cultural risk factors that are relevant to non-biological or non-medical trajectories of etiology, course, and treatment. These sociocultural analyses are consistent with health and disease research that uses social determinants of health models. The literature cited in Figure 2.1 is not all-inclusive, but it represents much of the seminal work done on dementia that features cultural factors.

We want to expand the understanding of dementia in Indigenous communities by using a more comprehensive perspective, one more closely aligned with the concept of "dementia syndrome" – the multiple inter-connecting, long-term factors (social, cultural, political, environmental, economic, and biological) that contribute to dementia. Dementia syndrome

FIGURE 2.1 Taxonomy of research on culture and dementia (selected)

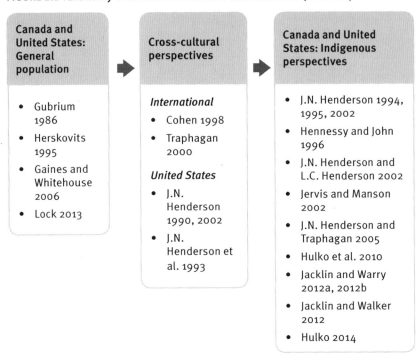

Canada and United States: General population	Cross-cultural perspectives	Canada and United States: Indigenous perspectives
• Gubrium 1986 • Herskovits 1995 • Gaines and Whitehouse 2006 • Lock 2013	*International* • Cohen 1998 • Traphagan 2000 *United States* • J.N. Henderson 1990, 2002 • J.N. Henderson et al. 1993	• J.N. Henderson 1994, 1995, 2002 • Hennessy and John 1996 • J.N. Henderson and L.C. Henderson 2002 • Jervis and Manson 2002 • J.N. Henderson and Traphagan 2005 • Hulko et al. 2010 • Jacklin and Warry 2012a, 2012b • Jacklin and Walker 2012 • Hulko 2014

is a "syndemic" condition that is a multifactorial causative web of biological, social, cultural, political, and economic inputs (Singer 2009). Dementia cannot be explained by genetics and biomedicine alone.[1] Although our main purpose is to capture the lived experience of dementia among Indigenous people, our model – which we call the Indigenous Syndemic Dementia Model (ISDM) – could be used to better understand dementia in all populations. Because we lack fully validated and supporting multifactorial and longitudinal prospective data for this method, our analysis here is best viewed as a hypothesis or road map for future research.

Models of Social and Biological Syntheses

Multifactorial concepts of disease etiology and course are now very common (Tesh 1988), if not universal. They reflect a variety of understandings. However, consider that two broad explanatory categories of disease causation and course are mainly used in typical contemporary scientific research, regardless of efforts to the contrary: the biomedical model, which privileges the biophysical environment as the primary cause of pathology, and the social determinants of disease model, which privileges the sociogenic sources that create health status, as is common in public health. As Charles Percy Snow (1959, 11) wrote long ago, however, "This polarization is sheer loss to us all."

In 1979, the medical sociologist Aaron Antonovsky compiled his life's work by conducting something of a self-meta-analysis. He identified the life factors that were broadly associated with "causing" good health. In his opinion, people who enjoyed good health possessed a "sense of coherence" about their lives. They saw their lives as characterized by psychosocial order, predictability, and rationality. The result was superior health status, compared to others who saw life as more chaotic and hostile.

The importance of Antonovsky's work on the sense of coherence was later confirmed by William Dressler and James Bindon (2000) in their study of "cultural consonance" and hypertension among African Americans who lived in rural Alabama. Other studies led by Dressler examined hypertension among Brazilians (Dressler, Balieiro, and Dos Santos 1998). In both locations, people experienced protection from hypertension if they perceived themselves and their life status to be appropriate for their age and circumstances. However, when there was a disjunction between their actual life experience and their desired life experience, the protection was reduced and the prevalence of hypertension was heightened. As an explanation for the presence or absence of hypertension, this effect was stronger than the socioeconomic status factors of income, occupation, and education.

The effects of a sense of coherence and cultural consonance are important to understand relative to the experience of Indigenous North Americans, whose lives have been disrupted by five hundred years of colonialism. The loss of a sense of coherence and the fragility of cultural consonance produce a high prevalence of stress-related conditions (Antonovsky 1979; Dressler, Balieiro, and Dos Santos 1998; Dressler and Bindon 2000). These include vascular dysfunction and associated connections to hypertension and metabolic disorders, resulting in heightened risk for cerebrovascular pathology. Overall, the effects of cumulative life stresses are indicated by the concept and term "allostatic load," referring to the effects of multiple life and biological stresses (Jackson, Knight, and Rafferty 2010; Peek et al. 2010) and are commonly found at high levels among non-majority populations.

Merrill Singer's (2009) Syndemic Model is an effort to bring the biomedical and social determinants of health models together as a comprehensive web of inputs that better explains health status dynamics. The Syndemic Model also posits that people are always partly healthy and partly diseased, so that no pristine condition of health can be attained. The "Mirage of

Health" (Dubos 1959) presages this concept and reinforces it, as does the nineteenth-century physician Rudolph Virchow's replacement of the "health" and/or "disease" dichotomy with the all-inclusive phrase that everyone lives in a constantly shifting state of "life under altered conditions" (cited in Rather 1958, 26; Nuland 1988, 305).

Multifactorial causal models include the Ecological Model, Social Ecology Model, Sociobiology Model, Biopsychosocial Model, and Syndemic Model. The Ecological Model is widely used to amplify the inclusion and consideration of multiple biological factors of disease causation and course so that the Doctrine of Specific Etiology and its contemporary extensions do not further limit scientific inquiry. As something of an addition to the Ecological Model, the Social Ecology Model is widely used to emphasize the inclusion of social determinants of health (Coreil, Bryant, and Henderson 2002).

In 1975, Edward O. Wilson published *Sociobiology: The New Synthesis*, which interdigitates genetics, biology, and human behaviour. Wilson saw sociobiology as an extension and explanation of natural selection, for which, however, altruistic behaviour seemed antithetical. Subsequent research showed how altruistic behavior could still favour one's representation of genes in the next generation.

The Biopsychosocial Model, as put forward by George Engle (1977), was intended to correct the limited Doctrine of Specific Etiology and the germ theory of disease. He added the word "culture" to a figure in a later essay (Engle 1980), but apparently it did not easily fit into the already clumsy "biopsychosocial" term.

Ann McElroy (1990) tried to better define the Biocultural Model. As the word "biocultural" suggests, there are two large components of input: biological factors, which include genetics, pathophysiology, specific diseases, and specific conditions; and cultural factors, which include beliefs, values, politics, and economics.

The Biocultural Model can exist in two basic forms (McElroy 1990). First is the "segmented" model. Here, the cultural and environmental data used to illuminate the biological data are delineated and sequentially ordered in segments. The result lacks interconnectedness, produces two parallel sets of findings, and suffers from linear thinking. Second is the "integrative" model, in which interconnections between the biological and sociocultural environments are emphasized.

Bioculturalism has been very well applied to diabetes by Dennis

Wiedman (2012) in his development of a Chronicities of Modernity Theory. Using an integrative biocultural perspective, he studied diabetes among the Kiowa, Comanche, and Apache of Oklahoma, knitting together many divergent threads to explain how the disease was the product of both endocrine system dysfunction and the cultural histories of people over long periods. If the biocultural effects are to be understood, the temporal dimension must be included. "Chronicities," as is found in his theory, are very explicitly markers of long-term exposure to noxious aspects of modern life.

In certain ways, the Indigenous Syndemic Dementia Model (ISDM) is similar to other multifactorial disease models. However, it avoids biomedical privilege (as subtly implied by "bio" being first in the word "biocultural"), though it fully includes biology as a key aspect of its explanation. ISDM also attempts to feature process analysis, by which multiple factors become operationalized and by which the non-biological becomes "biologized" (Singer 2009, 138–39). Most multifactorial models do not explain the process of "biologization," which leaves the biological and social factors or units conceptually adjacent but not commingled, as if there were no permeability of each putative "factor" boundary (see Jackson, Knight, and Rafferty 2010; Peek et al. 2010).

American Indian/Alaska Native Demographics

Until recently, most Indigenous people in the United States did not live long enough to exhibit a noticeable prevalence of dementia. Consequently, it was not seen as a serious problem for them or as really applying to them. Simply put, most did not reach the age of greatest risk for developing dementia symptoms, which is seventy-five and older (Administration on Aging 2014). Lifespan among the Indigenous populations of the United States has been and remains highly variable by location and accompanying situation. In some of the small and remote reservations, individuals do not live beyond their fifth decade. Although many Indigenous people in the United States do live longer than this, their lives as a group are shorter than those of the majority population.

According to the Administration on Aging (2014), an agency of the US Department of Health and Human Services, approximately 118,000 Indigenous people over the age of sixty-five resided in the United States in 1990; by 2010, that figure had risen to 235,000 (Figure 2.2). Projections to the year 2050 show that this group will approximately quadruple, reaching close to 1 million.

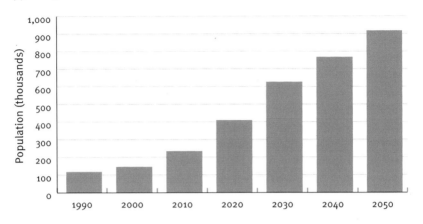

FIGURE 2.2 American Indian/Alaska Native population aged sixty-five and older, 1990–2050

The Indian Health Service of the United States uses age fifty-five as the threshold at which it considers an Indigenous person to be old. By contrast, the Administration on Aging uses age sixty-five as its threshold. Perhaps the Indian Health Service chose the younger age due to the phenomenon of accelerated aging, which can affect vulnerable populations that lead rigorous lives. The functional declines of age appear earlier for them than for those whose lives are less arduous. Using fifty-five as the threshold would greatly increase the number of people who are classed as "old" and the incidence of dementia that is associated with aging.

Indigenous Dementia: Cultural Factors

During the early 1990s, J. Neil Henderson conducted an in-service training session for a federally recognized tribe in the United States. Those who attended it were tribal community health representatives (CHRs) who had paraprofessional training in basic screening for blood pressure, glucose monitoring, and health resource information. A few minutes into the session, one CHR raised her hand, asked why it included dementia, and stated, "Indians don't get Alzheimer's disease." At the end of the forty-five-minute session, however, all the CHRs had thought of several of their older adult tribal clients who could potentially be diagnosed with some kind of dementia.

This incident is classic evidence of the potency of the cultural construction of disease. The CHRs had been working with people who showed signs of dementia but had not recognized them. Many probably assigned the symptoms to the normal and non-problematic category of "just old" and therefore not significant. However, at the end of the training session, after the signs and symptoms had been delineated, the participants' conceptual selectivity changed, and they became acutely aware of the presence of cognitive impairment among their clients.

In this section, we discuss a set of cultural factors that are salient to the development and course of dementia. Each factor operates in a specific life context that will vary across tribes and time. The factors examined here are tightly linked to Indigenous life in North America but are not a comprehensive list.

Of course, the lives of Indigenous people exhibit huge variations, and cultural heterogeneity is normally and fully present across and within tribes. Consequently, it is not possible to speak of effects that impinge equally on every individual of Indian Country. However, the cultural factors discussed below are of such magnitude that they would affect most of them.

Colonization Effects

Beginning several hundred years ago, European intrusion significantly disrupted the cultural and social organization of Indigenous people, whose lives still show the effects of this invasion. Such persistence is due in part to generational transmission of stories about the past and to the continuing bias against the Indigenous people of this continent, which is not well known by majority populations. The effects of colonization are ongoing and are indicated by shortened lifespan, excess morbidity and mortality, financial stress, and general health disparity (Gone and Trimble 2012). Nonetheless, the sheer fact that Indigenous people survived into the twenty-first century demonstrates tribal resilience and success.

If we apply the ideas of Antonovsky and Dressler, which argue that a sense of coherence and a perception of cultural consonance are linked with good health, we must recognize that the disruption of Indigenous life will result in the loss of coherence and consonance in daily social life and organization. As the products of this disruption, social and psychological pain and unvoiced stresses will have a negative impact on overall health. Health status, it is essential to note, includes not only physical health but emotional health as well. Suicide and substance abuse remain significant problems for many people in Indian Country (Brave Heart 2011; Gone and Trimble 2012). Likewise, its economic opportunities remain markedly underdeveloped despite government programs.

Poverty

Most people do not experience life at daily, extreme financial risk. However, poverty rates are higher among Indigenous people than for all other segments of society. For example, between 2007 and 2011, the American Indian and Alaska Native poverty rate ranged from 50.9 percent in Rapid City, South Dakota, to 16.6 percent in Anchorage, Alaska; the national all-populations rate during this period was 14.3 percent (US Census Bureau 2013). As is well known, poverty degrades all aspects of life, including health.

At first glance, it may seem obvious that the poor would have trouble making and attending appointments with health care providers and would therefore naturally experience higher levels of sickness. Though that is part of the story, the difficulty of staying healthy while living in poverty is due to many more factors than physician visits. Health status entails more than simply having a disease or not: it is the overall outcome of many elements of daily life over stretches of time. Poverty produces an ongoing sense of vulnerability, which is quite the opposite of a sense of coherence. Persistent anxieties, such as worrying about paying the bills and putting food on the table, trigger a flood of stress-related chemicals that are detrimental to health. Whereas everyone experiences stress at times, and occasionally extreme stress, a life of impoverishment involves the constant threat of collapse, a spectre that continually stimulates harmful stress responses.

Cultural Construct of Diabetes

Diabetes is a risk factor for dementia (see Chapter 7, this volume), making its cultural construction in Indian Country very pertinent. Cultural system disruption can be seen in the family dynamics of those who have the disease and in the biomedical providers' treatment of it. Linda Carson Henderson (2010) shows that American Indians who were diagnosed with diabetics often ignored the instructions on diet and physical activity that they received from their physician. If their medication were changed, some saw this as proof that the doctor was experimenting on them, and if it made them feel temporarily worse; some concluded that it was inappropriate or simply the result of incompetent medical treatment. Some declined to follow the instructions regarding diet and exercise because doing so would be seen as deviant behaviour in their own small community and family. Everyone wishes to be accepted and valued in his or her social group. In a resource-limited social environment, anyone who behaves very differently will typically be seen as refusing to follow accepted norms. Rejecting the status quo is a symbolic statement that one has allied with the authoritarian establishment. Consequently, obeying medical advice can be penalizing.

L.C. Henderson (2010) also shows that many providers do not take into account the wide range of acculturation among their American Indian patients. Although many understood that there were differences between "white Indians" (highly acculturated tribal members) and "Indian Indians" (adhering to many of the old cultural ways), it did not affect their practice and recommendations for treatment.

In summary, the pressures operating against adherence to primary and secondary preventive behaviours for diabetes originate within families and communities, and in attitudes regarding biomedical providers. American Indians who have diabetes find themselves in a social environment that seems almost tailor-made to prevent them from coping with the disease and mitigating its pathological effects.

Cultural Construct of Dementia

Beliefs held by people about what causes dementia and the nature of its course are highly variable. As noted earlier, some cultural constructs are based on biomedical precepts and may be perceived as sophisticated beliefs although not well demonstrated. Also, personal beliefs may be totally derived from non-scientific cultural belief systems. In today's world, the cultural constructs that attempt to explain dementia tend to blend lay biomedical perceptions with personal, culturally derived models.

A case study by J. Neil Henderson and Linda Carson Henderson (2002) dealt with a diabetic American Indian woman in her eighties who was living at home with her husband. She had severe cognitive impairment and an amputation below the knee due to her diabetes. She spent her days in a hospital bed that had been placed in her living room so that her caregivers could more easily attend to her. She was seen as ill-tempered and rude. One of her granddaughters was a tribal CHR who had received her in-service training from Neil Henderson. She took on the task of explaining to family and friends that the grandmother's behaviour was consistent with dementia. She intended to protect her from also losing her reputation as a kind, loving woman.

Hallucinations were also part of the grandmother's symptoms. She would sit in bed and chat with unseen others, pausing for their responses and conducting what would appear to be a two-sided conversation. Sometimes she looked out the window and said that she could see her parents in their garden; she identified favourite horses and pet dogs that were visible only to her; and she delivered a general report on what was going on outside.

In explaining this behaviour, the granddaughter said, "Pokni ['grandmother' in her native language] sees things that we don't." Significantly, she did not say, "Pokni sees things that aren't there." In fact, her wording reflected a cultural belief that the grandmother was not experiencing hallucinations due to brain pathology – she was communicating with people and circumstances on the "other side" prior to her own death. This is a case in which the biomedical nosology of dementia symptoms includes one that is singled out for special interpretation. The family saw the conversations with the other side as valuable. In their house, an older adult was revealing, in bits and pieces, that there was an other side after this life and that it was filled with recognizable people, animals, and places. To be sure, no one enjoyed her debility or her cutting comments, but one aspect of her dementia was interpreted in a way that was entirely positive.

North American Indigenous Dementia: Biology

Because dementia is, in part, a physical disease, genetics can reasonably be expected to play an important role in its analysis. At the sociocultural level, definitional criteria for labelling human groups based on distinctive behavioural features would be required not to confuse race or ethnicity labels with actual affinity groups. It is clear that such labelling is a completely cultural construct. Creating definitions of human groups by using biological or sociocultural data alone is destined to produce inaccuracies. From a biological perspective, most people are an amalgam, an admixture of genetic material that can originate in many diverse populations. Among American Indians, those who are classified as "full-bloods" may have less than 100 percent Indigenous genes. On the other hand, those who are socially classified as having 100 percent Indigenous genes may have a much smaller genetic load. Examples are easy to come by. For instance, to bolster their supply of males, which had diminished due to warfare, some Native people raided Anglo families and stole their children. None of the children had any Indigenous genes, yet they absorbed the tribal culture as they grew up (Namias 1993).

Biological factors related to the risk for dementia include genetic admixture. "Admixture" typically refers to the mingling of European genes with Indigenous North American genes. However, in the southeastern

United States particularly, there can be significant admixture among American Indians with persons of African descent. Ultimately, the genetic load, in terms of the proportion of Indigenous genes to those from other sources, can probably influence the frequency of the Apolipoprotein-Epsilon 4 allele, whether in homozygous or heterozygous conditions. In so doing, it can alter the risk for developing Alzheimer's disease. Genetic admixture can also influence the presence of alleles that control PPP1R3 (Hegele et al. 1998) and FAB P2 (Weiss et al. 2002), two genes that can disrupt metabolic function and influence hyperglycemia, hyperinsulinemia, and dyslipidemia.

The high prevalence of hypertension cannot be ignored as a factor related to the development of vascular pathology, with additional specificity to strokes. Likewise, smoking, atrial fibrillation, and general cardiovascular disease all predispose to vascular pathology and associated risk for strokes and resultant vascular dementia. Vascular dementia is a condition in which brain cells are killed by a stroke-like process, whereas Alzheimer's-type dementia kills brain cells through chemical pathways. Both destroy brain cells, though they do it in different ways.

One of the earliest medical studies of dementia among North American Indigenous people was undertaken by H.C. Hendrie et al. (1993). This study involved a Cree population southwest of Hudson Bay. The sample consisted of 192 Cree adults aged sixty-five and older. This early study was by no means a diagnostic one. It was an opportunistic short screening survey, which included a comparison to the Caucasian population of Winnipeg, Canada.

The results showed that eight of the Cree older adults had some form of dementia. Of these, one had Alzheimer's, four had multi-infarct dementia, two had alcohol dementia, and one had uncontrolled epilepsy combined with chronic alcoholism. The prevalence of Alzheimer's disease in this Cree sample was 0.5 percent. In Winnipeg's Caucasian population, the prevalence was 3.5 percent. The prevalence of dementia among the Cree was 4.2 percent, which matched that of Winnipeg.

It is important to understand the distinction between Alzheimer's disease and dementia. Whereas Alzheimer's must fit the cognitive assessment criteria noted above, "dementia" was used to indicate cognitive impairment due to other factors (Hendrie et al. 1993). These were probably related to vascular pathology and possibly to other types of less common dementia.

Roger Rosenberg et al. conducted another study among the Oklahoma Cherokee in 1996. In the Cherokee study, there were twenty-six cases and twenty-six controls. A major finding was an inverse relationship between the prevalence of Alzheimer's disease and the degree of genetic admixture of the individuals. The presence of the Apolipoprotein-E4 was not related to this finding.

In a study by J. Neil Henderson et al. (2002), a non-probability sample of Oklahoma Choctaw subjects was assessed for the presence of Apolipoprotein-E variation in the frequency of alleles 1–4. The presence of E4 alleles is associated with heightened risk for Alzheimer's (Liu et al. 2013). Permission for the study was given by the tribal council. CHRs of the tribe assisted in the recruitment of participants and were given in-service training on the topic of dementia recognition. The authors recruited 131 subjects by conducting a "question and answer" session at senior meal sites operated by the tribe and by asking licensed health care providers of the tribe to assist with selecting possible candidates. The CHRs also identified potential participants from their own client list. Blood samples were taken to determine the subjects' Apolipoprotein-E allele genotype.

The overall results of the study showed an inverse relationship between E4 allele frequency and the amount of Indigenous genes. More specifically, the frequency of the E4 allele was 6 percent in those who had a total loading of Indigenous genes (i.e., full-bloods), whereas it was 15 percent in the general white population. Due to the large range of genetic mixing in contemporary American Indians, sample stratification was necessary in accordance with degree of genetic admixture. In this sample, genetic load stratification showed that the frequency of the E4 allele varied in correspondence to genetic admixture. For subjects who possessed 50 to 100 percent of North American Indigenous genes, the frequency of the E4 allele was 6 percent. However, for those who had less than 50 percent, the frequency increased to match that of the Caucasian control group at 15 percent.

These few exploratory studies do not prove that North American Indigenous people have less risk or actual prevalence of Alzheimer's-type or vascular dementia. However, there is a thread of consistency across the Canadian Cree, the Oklahoma Cherokee, and Oklahoma Choctaw research participants in the apparent low prevalence of Alzheimer's-type dementia and a low frequency of the E4 allele. These data suggest that, compared to the majority white population, North American Indigenous peoples may have less genetic pressure toward Alzheimer's-type dementia.

The fact that "dementia" is a broad term that covers many types of organic brain disease raises the question of exactly what form is involved.

Though there are many types, one of the more frequent is vascular dementia. Its common risk factors include diabetes, hypertension, obesity, smoking, and alcohol abuse. Unfortunately, these are highly prevalent among North American Indigenous populations (Centers for Disease Control and Prevention 2011). Logic suggests that Indigenous people may be more at risk for vascular dementia and less at risk for Alzheimer's-type dementia. This differs from the epidemiologic profile for the majority population, in which Alzheimer's is most common, and vascular dementia is second. Analysis of brain tissue from dementia cases also shows that it is very common to have multiple pathologies in which the brain shows characteristic biomarkers of amyloid and vascular pathology (van Rossum et al. 2012).

Additional factors relating to North American Indigenous people and dementia include a number of diseases and pathological conditions. First are the risks for cardiovascular disease, including hypertension and atrial fibrillation. Combined with smoking, these are risk factors for stroke. Also, the high prevalence of diabetes mellitus in this population contributes to cardiovascular disease through conditions of hyperglycemia, hyperinsulinemia, and dyslipidemia. Moreover, type 2 diabetes is associated with vascular dementia but not with Alzheimer's neuropathology (Abner et al. 2016). These cardiovascular conditions and diabetes, particularly when present as co-morbid conditions, increase the risk of stroke. In turn, there is an increased risk over time for vascular dementia and its associated cognitive impairments, especially because growing numbers of North American Indigenous people are now living to the age of greatest risk.

An Indigenous Syndemic Model of Dementia

Formulating the Indigenous Syndemic Dementia Model to animate the possible combinations of effects that can result in dementia requires the creation of a hypothetical case. This case will be based on general and broad assumptions about the effects that would occur in real life. As stated earlier, the ISDM is a hypothesis-generating exercise, not a definitive proof. Stephen Kunitz (2007) points out that though the social determinants of health are very probably operating, direct proofs are lacking. Still, efforts to coalesce biological and social factors should provide better targets for intervention and research beyond a perpetual quest for a "pill cure" (Lock 2013; Lock and Nguyen 2010; Mendenhall 2012; Singer 2009; Wiedman 2012).

Creation of a hypothetical case requires that we consider age, gender, current medical conditions, lifestyle, acculturation status, and more. Because not every permutation of these characteristics can be presented here, we have chosen to build the hypothetical case around a man who is seventy-five years old and who has spent his life on a remote reservation in the United States. He speaks some of his native language, smokes, and has worked off-reservation alongside white people in blue-collar, labour-intensive agricultural, ranching, and forestry jobs. His family and peers consider him to be a "full-blood," and he participates in the religious and ceremonial life of his tribe. For convenience, we have named him Joseph.

Cognitive assessment would show that Joseph has a moderate degree of memory and thinking-skills loss. How did his late-life dementia come to be? Figure 2.3 maps important factors in Joseph's life – and in that of many Indigenous Americans. On their own, none of them would produce vascular dementia, but when operating dynamically and chronically over the lifespan, they could increase the probability that Joseph would develop the condition in old age.

FIGURE 2.3 Indigenous Syndemic Dementia Model for American Indians and Alaska Natives

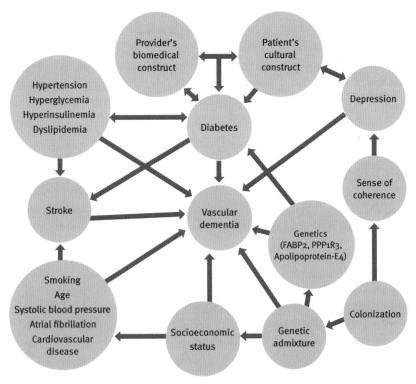

From the brief description of Joseph's history, one would expect that colonial disruptions of his life would be apparent every day, simply because he lives in the separate physical and social container that is called a reservation. Although reservation life can have positive aspects, such as supportive connections with kin and friends, its negative elements can operate even at very subtle levels. A reservation is a type of colonially created marker of social differentiation. It communicates that its inhabitants are different, that they don't fit in, that they are not encouraged to mix with the majority population, and that their destiny is controlled by the larger group. Joseph is old enough to have attended boarding school and has probably heard stories about these schools. Though some Native people recall them as a very positive life opportunity, many do not.

Joseph probably grew up with a very real perception of threats to his integrity. In the last several decades, telephone, radio, TV, CDs, and DVDs have all provided windows into the world outside the reservation. The disjunction between Joseph's life and the media's unending sales pitches for merchandise and life-fantasies in today's commerce-crazed society is easily imagined.

Low socioeconomic status is often associated with being marked as different and undesirable. By-products of a resource-deficient life include diminished overall health status, work in hazardous occupations, resultant physical traumas and exposure to toxic industrial chemicals, the use of tobacco and alcohol to mitigate stress, and the high consumption of cheap "comfort food," all collectively deleterious to health.

A low sense of coherence could be a constant theme of Joseph's life. Living with numerous and persistent losses of one's goals and self-destiny may well increase the likelihood of experiencing depression. Many elements of life are impaired by depression, including diabetes. It is useful to remember that sadness is only one feature of depression. Other important symptoms include sleep and appetite disruption, lack of concentration, and paralysis of will. Singly or collectively, these would probably interfere with Joseph's management of his own health or chronic diseases and his performance at work. They could also increase his risk of suicide.

All these factors could heighten Joseph's chances of developing diabetes. Among Indigenous people, this disease can be linked with genetics, but genes are probably not its main cause. Diabetes has systemic effects. It can literally weaken small blood vessels and can significantly damage certain parts of the body. For example, Joseph might have amputations of toes, fingers, or even the leg below the knee due to peripheral artery disease. His vision and his kidneys could be affected. And the damage to his blood vessels could diminish the supply of blood, nutrients, and oxygen to his brain.

Vascular dementia is the result of thousands of small bleeds in the brain to the extent that cognitive function is impaired. Though it is certainly unproven, research done by Rosenberg et al. (1996) and J.N. Henderson et al. (2002) suggests that Joseph may be more likely to develop vascular dementia than Alzheimer's-type dementia. This is because his life is characterized by numerous risk factors for stroke, whereas the Apolipoprotein-E4 allele that is associated with Alzheimer's disease is very probably not part of his genetic makeup.

At age seventy-five, Joseph has had long-term and significant exposure to the harmful effects of time. As Dennis Wiedman (2012) shows, chronicity of factors and events in a person's life is one of the keys that converts experiences into diseases and conditions, thereby increasing their allostatic load (Peek et al. 2010). This process may well be primarily the result of chronic stress. As James Jackson, Katherine Knight, and Jane Rafferty (2010) reveal, risky behaviour, including smoking, drinking, reckless driving, and other dangerous activities, along with eating large amounts of carbohydrate-rich foods, affects the hypothalamus-pituitary-adrenal cortex axis by producing cortisol, which then operates in a feedback system to damage blood vessels. In turn, it is easy to see the link between exacerbations of chronic stress and metabolic syndrome or full diabetes.

Although some Native people refer to diabetes as a "white man's disease," it is on the rise in their communities, which increases Joseph's chances of developing it. If he does, he may not adhere to the recommendations for its management. Eating well could be prohibitively expensive for him, and as mentioned above, following his doctor's instructions could alienate him from his social group. Furthermore, if Joseph's doctors do not understand that he sees the world in traditional Native terms, they may not provide information about diabetes and its management in ways that make sense to him. Medical professionals are constantly frustrated by diabetic patients who do not follow recommended management techniques. However, when doctors deal with Indigenous people, they must speak a language that accords with their patients' personal understanding of their condition, their lifestyle, and their maintenance of dignity.

❖ ❖ ❖

In summary, the Indigenous Syndemic Dementia Model provides a perspective in which late-life vascular dementia can be linked to a wide range of environmental conditions. The Indigenous people of Canada and the United States broadly share colonial histories that have generated the biological and social elements that literally embody their specific life experiences. Indigenous people in other parts of the globe probably experience similar colonial effects. Unfortunately, one particularly noxious embodiment for Indigenous people may be vascular dementia, from which individuals, families, and communities may struggle for years. Reducing its prevalence may be possible by preventive interventions such as the Healthy Brain Initiative (Centers for Disease Control 2014) and using the ISDM as a road map to identify macro and micro life experiences culminating in brain failure and cognitive separation from full enjoyment of later life.

Note

1   In reference to syndemic-type analysis, Edward Wilson (1998, 149) writes, "For its implications throughout biology and the social sciences, no subject is intellectually more important."

References

Abner, E.L., et al. 2016. "Diabetes Is Associated with Cerebrovascular but Not Alzheimer Neuropathology." *Alzheimer's and Dementia* 12: 882–89.

Administration on Aging. 2014. "Aging Statistics." https://www.acl.gov/sites/default/files/Aging%20and%20Disability%20in%20America/2014-Profile.pdf.

Antonovsky, Aaron. 1979. *Health, Stress, and Coping.* San Francisco: Jossey-Bass.

Brave Heart, Maria Yellow Horse. 2011. "The Historical Trauma Response among Natives and Its Relationship with Substance Abuse: A Lakota Illustration." *Journal of Psychoactive Drugs* 43: 282–90.

Centers for Disease Control and Prevention. 2011. *National Diabetes Fact Sheet: National Estimates and General Information on Diabetes and Prediabetes in the United States, 2011.* Atlanta: US Department of Health and Human Services.

–. 2014. "Healthy Brain Initiative." http://www.cdc.gov/aging/healthybrain/.

Cohen, Lawrence. 1998. *No Aging in India.* Berkeley: University of California Press.

Coreil, Jeannine, Carol Bryant, and J. Neil Henderson. 2002. "The Social Environment and Health." In *Social and Behavioral Foundations of Public Health,* ed. Jeannine Coreil, Carol Bryant, and J. Neil Henderson, 103–26. Thousand Oaks, CA: Sage.

Dressler, William W., Mauro Campos Balieiro, and Jose Ernesto Dos Santos. 1998. "Culture, Socioeconomic Status, and Physical and Mental Health in Brazil." *Medical Anthropology Quarterly* 12 (4): 424–46.

Dressler, William W., and James R. Bindon. 2000. "The Health Consequences of Cultural Consonance: Cultural Dimensions of Lifestyle, Social Support, and Arterial Blood Pressure in an African American community." *American Anthropologist* 102: 244–60.

Dubos, René. 1959. *Mirage of Health: Utopia, Progress, and Biological Change.* New York: Doubleday.

Engle, George L. 1977. "The Need for a New Medical Model: A Challenge for Biomedicine." *Science* 196: 129–36.

—. 1980. "The Clinical Application of the Biopsychosocial Model." *American Journal of Psychiatry* 137: 535–44.

Gaines, Atwood D., and Peter J. Whitehouse. 2006. "Building a Mystery: Alzheimer's Disease, Mild Cognitive Impairment, and Beyond." *Philosophy, Psychiatry, and Psychology* 13: 61–74.

Gone, Joseph P., and Joseph E. Trimble. 2012. "American Indian and Alaska Native Mental Health: Diverse Perspectives on Enduring Disparities." *Annual Review of Clinical Psychology* 8: 131–60.

Gubrium, Jaber. 1986. *Oldtimers and Alzheimer's: The Descriptive Organization of Senility.* Greenwich: JAI Press.

Hegele, Robert A., Stewart B. Harris, Bernard Zinman, Jian Wang, Henian Cao, Anthony J.G. Hanley, Lap-Chee Tsui, and Stephen W. Scherer. 1998. "Variation in the AU(AT)-Rich Element within the 3′-Untranslated Region of PPP1R3 Is Associated with Variation in Plasma Glucose in Aboriginal Canadians." *Journal of Clinical Endocrinology and Metabolism* 83: 3980–83.

Henderson, J. Neil. 1990. "Alzheimer's Disease in Cultural Context." In *Cultural Context of Aging: Worldwide Perspectives,* ed. J. Sokolosky, 315–30. New York: Bergin and Garvey.

—. 1994, November. "The Gerontology of American Indian Epidemiology." Paper presented at the American Public Health Association, Washington, DC.

—. 1995, June. "Biocultural Aspects of Dementia in Indian Country." Paper presented at American Indian Elders conference, National Resource Center on Native American Aging, Grand Forks, ND.

—. 2002. "The Experience and Interpretation of Dementia: Cross-Cultural Perspectives." *Journal of Cross-Cultural Gerontology* 17 (3): 195–96.

Henderson, J. Neil, Richard Crook, Julia Crook, John Hardy, Luisa Onstead, L. Carson Henderson, Pat Mayer, Bea Parker, Ronald Petersen, and Birdie Williams. 2002. "Apolipoprotein E4 and Tau Allele Frequencies among Choctaw Indians." *Neuroscience Letters* 324 (1): 77–79.

Henderson, J. Neil, M. Gutierrez-Mayka, J. Garcia, and S. Boyd. 1993. "A Model for Alzheimer's Disease Support Group Development in African-American and Hispanic Populations." *Gerontologist* 33: 409–14.

Henderson, J. Neil, and L. Carson Henderson. 2002. "Cultural Construction of Disease: A 'Supernormal' Construct of Dementia in an American Indian Tribe." *Journal of Cross-Cultural Gerontology* 17 (3): 197–212.

Henderson, J. Neil, and John W. Traphagan. 2005. "Cultural Factors in Dementia: Perspectives from the Anthropology of Aging." *Alzheimer Disease and Associated Disorders* 19 (4): 272–74.

Henderson, L. Carson. 2010. "Divergent Models of Diabetes among American Indian Elders." *Journal of Cross-Cultural Gerontology* 25 (4): 303–16.

Hendrie, H.C., et al. 1993. "Alzheimer's Disease Is Rare in Cree." *International Psychogeriatrics* 5 (1): 5–14.

Hennessy, Catherine Hagan, and Robert John. 1996. "American Indian Family Caregivers' Perceptions of Burden and Needed Support Services." *Journal of Applied Gerontology* 15 (3): 275–93.

Herskovits, Elizabeth. 1995. "Struggling over Subjectivity: Debates about the 'Self' and Alzheimer's Disease." *Medical Anthropology Quarterly* 9 (2): 146–64.

Hulko, Wendy. 2014. "Digging Up the Roots: Nature and Dementia for First Nation Elders." In *Creating Culturally Appropriate Outside Spaces and Experiences for People with Dementia,* ed. M. Marshall and J. Gilliard, 96–104. London: Jessica Kingsley.

Hulko, Wendy, Evelyn Camille, Elisabeth Antifeau, Mike Arnouse, Nicole Bachynski, and Denise Taylor. 2010. "Views of First Nation Elders on Memory Loss and Memory Care in Later Life." *Journal of Cross-Cultural Gerontology* 25 (4): 317–42.

Jacklin, Kristen, and Jennifer Walker. 2012. "Trends in Alzheimer's Disease and Related Dementias among First Nations and Inuit." Prepared for Health Canada, First Nations and Inuit Health, Home and Community Care Program.

Jacklin, Kristen, and Wayne Warry. 2012a. "Forgetting and Forgotten: Dementia in Aboriginal Seniors." *Anthropology and Aging Quarterly* 33: 13.

–. 2012b. "'They Knew Who She Was': Toward an Understanding of Diagnosis and Care of People with Dementia in Aboriginal Communities." *Alzheimer's and Dementia* 8 (4, suppl.): P431. DOI:10.1016/j.jalz.2012.05.1151.

Jackson, James S., Katherine M. Knight, and Jane A. Rafferty. 2010. "Race and Unhealthy Behaviors: Chronic Stress, the HPA Axis, and Physical and Mental Health Disparities over the Life Course." *American Journal of Public Health* 100: 933–40.

Jervis, Lori L., and Spero M. Manson. 2002. "American Indians/Alaska Natives and Dementia." *Alzheimer Disease and Associated Disorders* 16 (suppl. 2): S89–S95.

Kunitz, Stephen J. 2007. *The Health of Populations: General Theories and Particular Realities.* New York: Oxford University Press.

Liu, Chia-Chin, Takahisa Kanekiyo, Huaxi Xu, and Guojun Bu. 2013. "Apolipoprotein E and Alzheimer Disease: Risk, Mechanisms and Therapy." *Nature Reviews Neurology* 9: 106–18.

Lock, Margaret. 2013. *The Alzheimer Conundrum.* Princeton: Princeton University Press.

Lock, Margaret, and Vinh-Kim Nguyen. 2010. *An Anthropology of Biomedicine.* San Francisco: John Wiley and Sons.

McElroy, Ann. 1990. "Biocultural Models in Studies of Human Health and Adaptation." *Medical Anthropology Quarterly* 4 (3): 243–65.

Mendenhall, Emily. 2012 *Syndemic Suffering.* Walnut Creek: Left Coast Press.

Namias, June. 1993. *White Captives: Gender and Ethnicity on the American Frontier.* Chapel Hill: University of North Carolina Press.

Nuland, Sherwin B. 1988. *Doctors: The Biography of Medicine.* New York: Random House.

Peek, M. Kristen, Malcolm P. Cutchin, Jennifer J. Salinas, Kristen M. Sheffield, Karl Eschbach, Raymond P. Stowe, and James S. Goodwin. 2010. "Allostatic Load among Non-Hispanic Whites and Non-Hispanic Blacks, and People of Mexican Origin: Effects of Ethnicity, Nativity, and Acculturation." *American Journal of Public Health* 100: 940–46.

Rather, Lelland. 1958. *Disease, Life, and Man: Selected Essays.* Stanford, CA: Stanford University Press.

Rosenberg, Roger N., et al., 1996. "Genetic Factors for the Development of Alzheimer Disease in the Cherokee Indian." *Neurology* 53: 997–1000.

Singer, Merrill. 2009. *Introduction to Syndemics: A Critical Systems Approach to Public and Community Health.* San Francisco: John Wiley and Sons.

Snow, Charles Percy. 1959. *The Two Cultures and the Scientific Revolution: The Rede Lecture.* Cambridge: Cambridge University Press.

Tesh, Sylvia Noble. 1988. *Hidden Arguments: Political Ideology and Disease Prevention Policy.* New Brunswick, NJ: Rutgers University Press.

Traphagan, John. 2000. *Taming Oblivion: Aging Bodies and the Fear of Senility in Japan.* New York: State University of New York Press.

US Census Bureau. 2013, February 20. "American Indian and Alaska Native Poverty Rate About 50 Percent in Rapid City, S.D., and About 30 Percent in Five Other Cities, Census Bureau Reports." News release. https://www.census.gov/newsroom/press-releases/2013/cb13-29.html.

van Rossum, Ineke A., et al., 2012. "Injury Markers Predict Time to Dementia in Subjects with MCI and Amyloid Pathology." *Neurology* 79: 1809–16.

Weiss, Edward P., Michael D. Brown, Alan R. Shuldiner, and James M. Hagberg. 2002. "Fatty Acid Binding Protein-2 Gene Variants and Insulin Resistance: Gene and Gene-Environment Interaction Effects." *Physiological Genomics* 1: 145–57.

Wiedman, Dennis. 2012. "Native American Embodiment of the Chronicities of Modernity: Reservation Food, Diabetes, and the Metabolic Syndrome among the Kiowa, Comanche, and Apache." *Medical Anthropology Quarterly* 26 (4): 595–613.

Wilson, Edward O. 1975. *Sociobiology: The New Synthesis.* Cambridge, MA: Harvard University Press.

–. 1998. *Consilience: The Unity of Knowledge.* New York: Knopf.

CHAPTER 3

A STORY ABOUT JOE IN THE NEWS MEDIA
Decolonizing Dementia Discourse

Suzanne MacLeod

Alzheimer's sufferer sits in remand.

— KUSCH (2010B)

Alzheimer's patient CHARGED.

— SANDERS AND PAUL (2011)

WHEN JOE MCLEOD MADE the headlines in Winnipeg and across Canada, only part of his story was told. It focused on his Alzheimer's disease – a form of dementia – and his related violent behaviours that twice landed him in jail. The first time was for pushing his wife, who needed stitches, and the second time was for pushing a fellow resident in long-term care, Frank Alexander, who later died from his injuries. According to the media, Joe's story was a "tragic microcosm" of the "Alzheimer's crisis" that is expected to mushroom in Canada as the population ages ("Our Alzheimer's Crisis" 2013). Canada has a shortage of long-term-care beds (Rockwood and Keren 2010, 876), which are often needed by people who exhibit dementia-related violent behaviours – also understood as responsive behaviours reflecting "unmet needs" (Cohen-Mansfield et al. 2010, 1459; Smith and Buckwalter

2005, 40). One headline about Joe read, "We Need a Dementia Strategy, Not Grandpa Prisons" (Picard 2010, L5).

However, what the news media typically did not mention was that Joe and his wife had been forced to leave their home on the Pine Creek Reserve to access dementia care services in Winnipeg. Joe's indigeneity was noted only twice in twenty-four articles, and the press failed to discuss the colonial context of both his experiences and the dementia crisis discourse. Instead, a national "amnesia" (Anderson and Robertson 2011; Harding 2006; Tuck and Fine 2007), or "cult of forgetfulness" (Stanner 1979, 214), persisted in its coverage. As a result, Canada's ongoing colonial legacy – in health care and beyond – was forgotten. Indeed, the crisis focus dominates public discourse and prevents possibilities for more reflective and critical conversations, including subjugated discourses about dementia and dementia care. This concerns me as a "white" fourth-generation settler of British descent who is currently employed as a social worker in dementia care. Thus, I employ a decolonizing lens in conducting a poststructural discourse analysis of the media depiction of Joe and his needs for care.

Colonialism and Health Care in Canada

To complicate my settler lens on Joe's experiences, I conducted a review of multiple literatures. Among these were works that discussed colonialism in Canada – identified by some as "genocide" (Chrisjohn and Young 2006, 60) – and ongoing colonialism in Canada's health care system. This literature identified health disparities between Indigenous and non-Indigenous persons (Czyzewski 2011; Lavoie 2004) as well as federal-provincial jurisdiction and funding barriers to Indigenous health (Beatty and Berdahl 2011; Fiske and Browne 2006; Kelly 2011; Lavoie 2004; Lavoie, Forget, and Browne 2010). Karina Czyzewski (2011, 10) explains that a colonial legacy undergirds such disparities in and barriers to Indigenous health:

> If an Indigenous [social determinants of health] framework demonstrates that settler ideologies, interactions and imposed systems are a significant cause of the causes of Indigenous ill-health, then settlers need to confront the persistence of racist attitudes and with this, society's role, along with the state and its institutions, at contributing to poor health outcomes.

My analysis unsettles the persistence of racist attitudes about dementia and health care – my own and those of institutions such as the mainstream news media. Importantly, dementia has been considered a new phenomenon in Indigenous communities, related not to disease but to colonization and social factors (Hulko et al. 2010, 324, 327). Shawnda Lanting et al. (2011) and Wendy Hulko et al. (2010) report that there is no word for "dementia" in the Indigenous languages of their research participants. Rather, Indigenous perspectives account for cognitive and behavioural changes as part of normal aging processes in a circular conception of the lifespan (Lanting et al. 2011, 103, 110). Indigenous people emphasize culturally grounded health care (Lanting et al. 2011, 103), "supporting one another," and "the well-being of communities and collective action to promote and maintain holistic health" (Hulko et al. 2010, 335).

Further, I contextualize Joe's story vis-à-vis the Canadian media and the justice system. Consequently, the following are taken into account: the over-representation of Indigenous persons in the criminal justice system (Bracken, Deane, and Morrissette 2009; Furniss 2001; Gebhard 2012; Van Herk, Smith, and Andrew 2011); portrayals of Indigenous people in the media (Furniss 2001; Harding 2006; Henry and Tator 2002); and settler colonial "amnesia" (Anderson and Robertson 2011; Tuck and Fine 2007; Harding 2006). For instance, regarding the depiction of Aboriginal people in Canadian news texts from the 1860s and the 1990s, Robert Harding (2006, 206) observes that the media devote "considerable attention to reporting on the extreme circumstances in which many contemporary aboriginal people live" but do not analyze the sociopolitical context of these living conditions or "the impact of Canada's long history of colonialism on aboriginal people."

Decolonizing Theoretical Approach

Writing from an Indigenous perspective, Margaret Kovach (2005, 21, 28, 33) states that decolonizing research, also known as "researching back," has the objectives of resistance, recovery, and renewal. It seems fitting, in a book about memory loss, that the process of decolonization involves researching back, which demands the collective remembering or, as Eve Tuck and Michelle Fine argue (2007, 155, emphasis in original), the "*un*forgetting" of ongoing colonialism. However, Taiaiake Alfred (1999, 143) reminds me that decolonization is not just about researching back or remembering, but also about taking back: "the time has come for people who are from someplace

Indian to take back the discourse on Indians." So how might my research from a white settler position support and complement Indigenous processes of taking back discourse? Clearly, my place is not to research Indigenous people. Instead, I turn the lens on my settler role in decolonization (Kovach 2005, 26) by identifying and taking apart the discourses, institutions, policies, and practices that, effectively in my name, "the colonizers erected in order to diminish and/or destroy Indigenous cultures and traditional ways of life" (Hulko et al. 2010, 320). To this end, I did not interview Joe, his family, or their Indigenous community or ask them to help with my research. Instead, I drew on Indigenous perspectives shared in academic literature to guide my interrogation of the newspaper articles. Leanne Simpson (2008, 14) states that "settler society must ... choose to change their ways, to decolonize their relationships with the land and Indigenous Nations, and to join with [Indigenous people] in building a sustainable future based upon mutual recognition, justice, and respect." My hope is that my research "disrupts settler colonialism" (Tuck and Yang 2012, 19) and contributes in a small way toward changing Indigenous-settler relationships in health care, by noticing and challenging taken-for-granted colonial and crisis-based discussions regarding "what to do" about dementia in Canada.

Poststructural Research

Disrupting Dominant Discourse

I draw upon poststructural methodology and its concepts of discourse and the politics of truth to perform a genealogical discourse analysis of the selected newspaper articles. According to poststructural thought, "reality" is a social construction that is produced and reflected through language and discourse (Bartlett and O'Connor 2010, 52). Discourses are "historically specific systems of meaning or ways of making sense of the world ... shaped by social practices and in turn shap[ing] social relationships and institutions" (Comack and Bowness 2010, 36). Discourses, then, have material effects that "specify what is morally, socially and legally un/acceptable at any given moment in time" (Carabine 2001, 274). Indeed, as Michel Foucault (1980, 131) argues, discourses produce knowledge and power, and some are more powerful than others: "Each society has its régime of truth, its 'general politics' of truth: that is, the types of discourse which it accepts and makes function as true." Poststructural discourse analysis attempts to "reveal discursive practices in their complexity and density" (Foucault 2011, 230).

Elizabeth Comack and Evan Bowness (2010, 46) demonstrate how this methodology can draw attention to counter-discourse, which, in naming inequality and centring Indigenous peoples, "holds the greatest potential for disrupting the dominant discourse." My analysis problematizes the dementia crisis discourse in the newspaper stories about Joe, both to illustrate colonial assumptions in dementia care and to support decolonizing approaches.

Data from the News Coverage

I examined Joe's story as presented in twenty-four articles and editorials published in the *Winnipeg Free Press,* the *Toronto Globe and Mail,* and the *Toronto National Post* to include both local and national perspectives on the case. Though newspapers across the country – from Kamloops to Ottawa – covered aspects of the story, I focused primarily on the *Winnipeg Free Press,* given its original, local coverage over the duration of the case. The selected articles begin with Joe's first incarceration for assaulting his wife (Kusch 2010e), move to his bail hearing for manslaughter after the death of Frank ("Local Alzheimer's Patient" 2011), and end with the initiation by the Government of Manitoba of an inquest into the case ("Our Alzheimer's Crisis" 2013).

Genealogical Discourse Analysis

I employed one approach to poststructural methodology called genealogical discourse analysis, which works to complete a history – or problematization – of the present (Koopman 2013, 17) by "rethink[ing] and call[ing] into question the given truths of our world" (Tamboukou 1999, 208). The news as offered in newspapers, for example, is understood to reflect, and create, "a particular view of reality" (Cheek 2000, 43). The genealogical researcher tries to consider a multiplicity of truths or perspectives by looking for absences and silences from the dominant discourses in the texts and considering resistances and counter-discourses (Carabine 2001, 281). Poststructural methodology assumes that all knowledge – and research – is localized and subjective. Thus, it eschews a formal method or particular "recipe" in favour of a more flexible, iterative, and intuitive process (Cheek 2000). That considered, I nonetheless implemented a "plan" to complete my analysis. First, I extensively reread the articles to "get an overall 'feel' for the data" (Carabine 2001, 283). In the analytical phase, I developed a table to track not only the details of the stories but also the speakers or sources, headlines, graphics, and repeated themes to detect overarching emphasis as well as gaps in the presentation of Joe's "problem" with dementia care and proposed solutions. Throughout this process, as contextual gaps or questions arose, I expanded my literature review to further consider Indigenous and decolonizing perspectives.

Discourses in the Media Coverage

The twenty-four newspaper articles were published in three clusters. The first two, consisting of twenty stories, date from the fall of 2010 and the spring and summer of 2011. They deal with Joe's first and second imprisonments. The third cluster, comprising only four articles, runs from February 2012 to March 2013. Two stories from February 2012 announce that Joe will not be tried for manslaughter (McIntyre 2012; "Winnipeg Man with Alzheimer's" 2012), and an editorial of January 2013 states that the Manitoba government has initiated "a full inquest into the homicide" of Frank Alexander ("Our Alzheimer's Crisis" 2013). In a March 2013 editorial, written after a resident was killed in a Toronto seniors' home, Joe's story is cited as an example of resident-to-resident violence in long-term care ("Our Growing Elder-Care Crisis" 2013).

Criminalization Discourse

The first cluster of articles focuses on the details of Joe's initial imprisonment in the Winnipeg Remand Centre and his subsequent transfer to a residential care facility. The criminalization discourse that pervades most of the articles is established immediately, and Joe is presented as a violent person whose dementia-related behaviour is better handled by police intervention and jail than by health care services. For example, the stories indicate that he has Alzheimer's disease and explain that he pushed his wife, Rose, in confusion. Not knowing where to turn, she called the police, feeling she "didn't have a choice" (Kusch 2010a) but to press domestic assault charges so that she and Joe could get help. The police took Joe to hospital, which then released him to the remand centre. According to Joe's son, Ron, "the police were just doing their job," but the journalist also stated that Ron "was surprised the doctors at Concordia released his dad" (Kusch 2010b). The articles repeatedly highlight that Rose needed stitches for her injuries, while also noting that she wanted the assault charges dropped. The emphasis on Joe's criminality continues in the second cluster of stories. These report that Joe pushed Frank Alexander at Parkview Place, the Winnipeg care home in which they lived, that Frank subsequently died due to his injuries, and that Joe was once again charged, this time with aggravated assault and later manslaughter, and placed in jail. The events leading to his previous imprisonment are retold throughout.

System Crisis Discourse

Overall, the articles state that Joe's story is a "unique case" (Kusch 2010b; Mitchell 2010) that shows "cracks" (Kusch 2010a; Mitchell 2010) and "failure" (Kusch 2010b; Picard 2010, L5) in the health care and justice systems. One early write-up, detailing Joe's first release from jail, suggests that his story became national news because it shone "a light on the challenges faced by medical and legal authorities in dealing with Alzheimer's sufferers" (Kusch 2010d). In the second cluster of articles, particularly in the national columns about Joe's second imprisonment, there is increased emphasis on presenting his case as an example of the "coming Alzheimer's crisis" (Gurney 2011a), given the aging of the population and the demands this will place on family caregivers and "an already over-burdened health care system" ("Long-Term Strategy" 2011). The reports suggest that "society must steel itself for the wave of Alzheimer's and dementia that is our future" (Gurney 2011a).

"Violent" Joe and "Innocent" Frank: (De)racializing Discourses

The media coverage presents Joe as an "aggressive Alzheimer's patient," whereas Frank is remembered as an "innocent person" (Sanders 2011; Sanders and Paul 2011), a Second World War veteran "who did us all proud" (O'Connor 2011). To all appearances, Frank is a white settler, and the news stories do not suggest otherwise. As Jo-Anne Fiske and Annette Browne (2006, 109) observe in their research about discourses that marginalize Aboriginal women vis-à-vis the health care system, when dominant discourses only identify the positionality of Aboriginal individuals, all other stakeholders are "implicitly disassociated from a minority culture and viewed as representing a dominant perspective that is couched in racial/gender/class neutrality." Joe, however, is subtly, but nonetheless clearly, racialized as an Indigenous person. He is only twice referred to as recently living on the Pine Creek Reserve, but his photo is displayed multiple times, so the reader comes to know him as an Indigenous man who is also violent. The discourse about his violent nature is emphasized by his juxtaposition with Frank. The press coverage typically notes that Joe is a married father and grandfather who is an "Alzheimer's sufferer" (Kusch 2010a, 2010b, 2010c), but only four articles give specific information about his personhood and belonging in community. For instance, these state that Joe is a retired CNR worker (Kusch 2010c; "Winnipeg Man with Alzheimer's" 2012) who cultivated a garden (Mitchell 2010), "loved rural life" (Martin 2011a), and "was active in [the Pine Creek] band government" (Martin 2011a). In contrast, Frank's navy service during the Second World War and his subsequent dry-cleaning career are mentioned seven times ("Long-Term Strategy" 2011; Martin 2011b; McIntyre 2012; O'Connor 2011; Sanders 2011; Sanders and Paul 2011; "Winnipeg Man with Alzheimer's" 2012), despite the fact that he appears in fewer articles than Joe.

What's Missing from the Dominant Discourses?

Although the newspaper articles do include some direct quotes from Joe's wife and children, the dominant voices are those of police officers, politicians, and health authority officials. Only one report explicitly articulates an Indigenous perspective on health care support for aging people. It covers a press conference held by the Southern Chiefs Organization, which included the chief from Joe's home community (Martin 2011a).

Unpacking and Resisting Colonial Amnesia

Overall, the articles about Joe's experiences with dementia care embody a national or colonial amnesia. This works to deny the history of the European colonization of North America and the "harrowing tale of decimation of the Indigenous population by infectious disease, warfare, and an active suppression of culture and identity" (Kirmayer, Brass, and Tait 2001, 6). The media coverage does not suggest that the settler population or the government should work toward justice for Indigenous peoples in areas such as treaty making, residential school healing, and self-government (Harding 2006, 231). By focusing primarily on Joe's story within the dominant discourse of the dementia care crisis, the press "*unhing[es]* the present from the past" and misses an opportunity to acknowledge and support the needs of Indigenous people and to deconstruct the barriers they experience to well-being and health care (Harding 2006, 206, emphasis in original).

Joe in Jail: Deconstructing Racist Stereotyping in the Media Coverage

According to Mark Anderson and Carmen Robertson (2011, 264), "a steady diet of bad news about Aboriginals is swallowed up as natural, even predictable." Furthermore, the association of Indigenous people "with violence and criminality is an argumentative ploy that has been used historically to discredit aboriginal people and causes in news discourse" (Harding 2006, 221). In relaying the "bad news" about Joe, the press seems to offer a sympathetic view on the "tragedy" (Martin 2011a) of his experience in a failing health system, at least on the surface. For example, the articles explain that persons with dementia are unable to form criminal intent (Gurney 2011c; O'Connor 2011; Paul 2011); that imprisoning someone with dementia is "appalling" and "unacceptable" (Kusch 2010b; Picard 2010, L5); that "care should never be dependent on criminal charges" (Picard 2010, L5); and that the "justice system is designed to rehabilitate and punish criminals, not warehouse the sick" (Gurney 2011c). However, at the same time, the police are not held responsible for their actions. After Frank was injured, they concluded that they had "no choice but to charge McLeod with assault," and in deciding what to do with "the accused," they determined "the best option was the Remand Centre" (Sanders and Paul 2011). These statements are presented as objective fact, with no critical analysis. Collectively, the accounts undermine Joe and deny his right to receive support in a health care organization.

Contemporary media discourse is sanitized of "blatant" racism, but it nonetheless employs slightly more subtle common-sense conventions to evoke and sustain the racist stereotyping of Indigenous people as violent criminals (Anderson and Robertson 2011, 267). Similarly, though two articles do mention that Joe was "a non-violent man before his illness" and "a gentle man in another life" (Gurney 2011b; O'Connor 2011), his peaceful humanity is lost in the overriding sensational discussion of his violence and criminality. The overall message is that Joe is "Mr. Alexander's killer" ("Our Alzheimer's Crisis" 2013). The newspaper reports evoke racist stereotyping by constructing him as someone who has a "history of violence" (O'Connor 2011), repeatedly "behind bars" and charged with "aggravated assault" (Paul 2011; Sanders and Paul 2011). This normalizes Joe as a man who is inherently "in trouble" with the law (O'Connor 2011). It legitimizes his treatment as a violent criminal, even though the same articles also assert that "clearly he is not capable of forming criminal intent" (Gurney 2011c) and quote the CEO of the Alzheimer Society of Manitoba as stating, "people with Alzheimer's disease often don't know what has happened, or even where they are. They are disoriented. They are confused – and there's not an intent. It's not a pre-meditative intent" (O'Connor 2011).

An Overwhelmed Health Care System and Over-Policing

The newspapers do occasionally disrupt the construction of Joe as threatening by explaining that hitting out in confusion is common dementia behaviour (Gurney 2011a, 2011b, 2011c; Paul 2011), but the overriding impression is that he is a violent criminal – and Indigenous. The headlines repeatedly declare his criminality by focusing on the charges against him and his imprisonments. Two reports even suggest that jail was the only safe place for him: he "had no safe place to be but jail" (Sanders 2011) and "was kept in jail for safety reasons" (McIntyre 2012). This discourse, in which jail provides safety for Joe, and presumably from Joe, is reinforced by the implication that he apparently had nowhere else to go. The write-ups emphasize that hospitals and long-term-care facilities are overflowing with the aging population (Gurney 2011c; "Our Alzheimer's Crisis" 2013), "a grey wave," as journalist Alexandra Paul (2011) puts it. They point out the extreme shortage of facilities "for those at risk of committing violence" such as "people like McLeod" (Gurney 2011c; Paul 2011). However, what's missing is a reminder that the Winnipeg Remand Centre "has been consistently over capacity for years" as well (CBC News 2012). The media coverage indicates that Joe's imprisonment for his dementia-related behaviour raises "disturbing concerns for health care that are national in scope" (Paul 2011), but its analysis stops at system failure. And though it poses questions – at least rhetorical ones – it does not attempt to answer them either critically or with a decolonizing lens. Writing for the *Winnipeg Free Press,* Catherine Mitchell (2010) states, "The system is showing its cracks. How else to explain how Joe McLeod was not listed as a candidate for emergency placement, but rather a man better suited to a holding cell?" And Larry Kusch (2010a) asks, "What's wrong with the system that somebody who's got Alzheimer's can end up in jail instead of in a proper care facility?"

The media analysis fails to consider the possibility that discriminatory racist practices by police and hospital staff might have made Joe "better suited to a holding cell" (Mitchell 2010). For example, according to Elizabeth Furniss (2001, 2), "widespread attitudes of racism on the part of non-Aboriginal society ... have led to the miscarriages of justice, [and] the over-policing of the Aboriginal population" based on the "presumption of the criminality of Aboriginal people." As a result, Indigenous people are disproportionately represented in the Canadian criminal justice system (Bracken, Deane, and Morrissette 2009, 65; Furniss 2001, 2; Van Herk, Smith, and Andrew 2011, 58). They make up 3 percent of the Canadian population but constitute 17 percent of the prison population (Bracken, Deane, and Morrissette 2009, 65; Gebhard 2012, 7). The news coverage constructs Joe's incarceration as an isolated example of a "cascade of unfortunate events" (Mitchell 2010) rather than a cascade of deeply embedded over-policing practices rooted in the colonial history of the health and justice systems. As a result, the reading public is encouraged to "remain unaware of and uncritical about the current state of Aboriginal/non-Aboriginal relations and the way in which ... racism, local prejudice, and chronic problems within the Canadian justice system [are] central and ongoing realities in the lives of Aboriginal people" (Furniss 2001, 26).

Resisting Joe's Assimilation into the Dementia Crisis Discourse

Except for one story, the media coverage – "whether by deliberate intent or by unconscious cultural habit" (Furniss 2001, 16) – overlooks Indigenous perspectives on health care for seniors. The news reports effectively assimilate Joe's experiences into the dominant discourse about the Alzheimer's crisis and the failure of a supposedly universal health care system to provide dementia care to an apparently homogeneous aging population. Harding (2006, 206) also observes that the dominant discourse resists the idea that Indigenous people have distinctive needs by promoting identical treatment for everyone: "The *active* biological racism of colonial times has given way to a passive and sanitized *ethnocentrism* characterized by a creed of 'identical treatment' which emphasizes equality of opportunity ... while denying the existence of contemporary racist practices, attitudes and outcomes" (emphasis in original). Similarly, in the reports on Joe's story, the overarching assumption is that one-size-fits-all national and provincial dementia strategies are needed to cope with the approaching "demographic tidal wave" that threatens provincial health budgets (Gurney 2011c; "Long-Term Strategy" 2011; Paul 2011; Picard 2010, L5). Clearly, a crisis discourse about dementia and dementia care has "taken hold in the minds of the public and policy-makers" (Gee and Gutman 2000, 2). That said, Ann Robertson (1991, 147) reminds us that we need not "believe ourselves to be at the mercy of blind forces, such as demographic and economic imperatives, as if these existed outside of the realm of public discussion and debate."

Just as it is important to problematize the discourse that presents dementia as a crisis and a socioeconomic threat, a decolonizing perspective demands that the media's settler bias on the "crisis" be critiqued as well. As Frances Henry and Carol Tator (2002, 226) observe, the "Canadian media so often construct a discursive sketch of Canadian society that silences, erases, and marginalizes a significant proportion of this country's population." Certainly, the needs of Joe and other Indigenous seniors are marginalized in the news coverage. Joe's story is decontextualized and framed as that of one individual who fell through the cracks in a flawed and overwhelmed system, not as an Indigenous man who was possibly up against racist stereotypes and colonial health care and justice systems. Joe's challenges are shifted "away from structures, processes and relations of power" (Fiske and Browne 2006, 98), even though it is well accepted that colonization is a social determinant of Indigenous health (Czyzewski 2011). The focus on a national dementia crisis neglects to acknowledge the history of Indigenous-settler relations and the unique status of Indigenous people within the colonial state. In doing so, it effectively contributes to continued health disparities between the Indigenous and non-Indigenous populations (Czyzewski 2011, 2, 3, 9).

Centring Indigenous Views on Solutions for Senior Care

Although one article did include Indigenous political perspectives on the experiences of Joe and Frank, its points were marginalized by the series of otherwise sensationalist reports focused on a national dementia crisis. Thus, as Harding (2006, 225) notes, its "impact is diluted." In this way, the "voices of aboriginal people are *selectively* incorporated into news discourse in ways that largely support the dominant frame" (Harding 2006, 225, emphasis in original). However, in an effort to make space for Indigenous counter-discourses and to consider the colonial context of Joe's experiences, I would like to closely examine this lone article. Titled "Caring for Reserves' Seniors: Tragedy Sparks Call to Provide for the Elderly on First Nations" (Martin 2011a), it was published in the spring of 2011, after Joe's second imprisonment, and it documents a press conference held by the Southern Chiefs Organization (SCO) in Manitoba. Clearly, the chiefs had to demand to be heard, as their perspectives were not otherwise included in the news reports. Chief Nepinak of Pine Creek First Nation, SCO Grand Chief Shannacappo, and Joe's daughter Faye are all quoted, but representatives from the involved police and health care institutions (who appear throughout the other coverage) are not. Yet again an opportunity is missed to encourage these authorities to reflect on Indigenous concerns and to be accountable for persistent colonial relations.

The chiefs express a "need to prepare" and find "new solutions to keep aging First Nations residents safe" (Martin 2011a). In calling for Indigenous-specific infrastructure and support for seniors, they disrupt the dominant discourse, which advocates for a national dementia strategy: "We want to keep our elders in the community and provide them with the support they need so that tragedies like this don't need to happen" (Nepinak quoted in Martin 2011a). More specifically, they highlight the inadequacy of on-reserve services. Whereas "only seven of Manitoba's 64 First Nations have long-term care facilities," the population of Indigenous seniors is "large enough to support more ... Pine Creek First Nation alone has 200 seniors" (Martin 2011a). In fact, Aboriginal seniors (aged fifty-five and older) constitute the most rapidly growing demographic group in Canada (Lanting et al. 2011, 104). Like many Indigenous seniors, however, Joe was forced to leave his home to try to access dementia care supports. The literature confirms that because of the lack of health care services in rural and northern communities, Indigenous seniors must travel to larger urban centres (Beatty and Berdahl 2011; Habjan, Prince, and Kelley 2012). In Winnipeg alone, the Aboriginal senior population grew by 40 percent between 2001 and 2006, whereas that of non-Aboriginal seniors increased by less than 4 percent (Beatty and Berdahl 2011, 3). And though urban institutions may meet the "medical needs" of Indigenous seniors, Belulah Beatty and Lolene Berdahl (2011, 8) note that this often comes at the expense of their "mental and cultural well-being." Josée Lavoie, Evelyn Forget, and Annette Browne (2010, 94) similarly contend that "even when individuals can find their way to off-reserve services ... research shows that tacit and overt discriminatory practices and policies continue to marginalize many First Nations individuals in the mainstream health care system."

In the news story, Chief Nepinak cites these barriers to Indigenous seniors' health and advocates that "developing new models of on-reserve care that combine medical support, cultural traditions and family and community networks could make for healthier seniors and better health outcomes" (Martin 2011a). He also states that Indigenous leaders "have long been working with government agencies to try working out a new solution for caring for First Nations seniors" (Martin 2011a). However, "jurisdictional push and pull has left a gap in care when it comes to long-term facilities" (Martin 2011a). Miranda Kelly (2011, 1) notes that the "disproportionate burdens of ill health experienced by First Nations have been attributed to an uncoordinated, fragmented health care system." Unfortunately, in the news article under examination, the jurisdictional gaps, fragmentation, and funding inequities are not specified or analyzed. Josephine Etowa, Charlotte Jesty, and Adele Vukic (2011, 31) write that there is a "tendency to gloss over inequities in health and health care ... instead of examining the influential and complex interplay of historical, socioeconomic and political forces." Currently, the federal government is responsible for funding First Nations health care on-reserve, and the provinces are responsible for primary health care service delivery off-reserve (Kelly 2011, 1). However, funding allocation to First Nations communities "does not reflect the actual population being served" (Lavoie 2004, 345) or the "identified level of need" (Habjan, Prince, and Kelley 2012, 218). Finally, Beatty and Berdahl's (2011, 1) research, which examines the health care challenges facing Aboriginal seniors in urban Canada, makes five policy recommendations to ameliorate the situation. These include establishing First Nations long-term-care facilities on-reserve and Aboriginal long-term-care facilities in major Prairie cities, as well as developing "culturally responsive programming and employment in health-care systems" (Beatty and Berdahl 2011, 10). Except for one news article, however, such Indigenous-specific health care infrastructure policy recommendations do not enter the dominant crisis discourse in the media coverage of Joe's life.

❖ ❖ ❖

With the stories, experiences, and legacies of colonialism that "float through all of us" (Tuck and Fine 2007, 146) – settler and Indigenous persons alike – even in the most basic aspects of aging and health care supports, the mainstream media coverage of Joe's story demonstrates that the "discursive reproduction of racism reinforces the power of the dominant culture and legitimizes systems of inequality" (Henry and Tator 2002, 13). If we are to decolonize such deeply ingrained inequality, we must remember colonization: "It is important to contextualize and speak of colonial policies and the legacies they left behind when speaking about Indigenous mental health, and the health disparities we see when compared to the mainstream population" (Czyzewski 2011, 8). Furthermore, the Indigenous social determinants of health framework demonstrates that we must also speak of, and actively support, Indigenous governance and land rights to generate the cultural, social, and economic conditions that improve physical, mental, emotional, and spiritual health (Czyzewski 2011, 10).

Finally, as stories about persons with dementia, the challenges of their care, and dementia-related behaviours continue to hit the news, further research and calm conversation are clearly needed to imagine creative and compassionate ways to meet the needs of people with dementia and keep them out of jail. However, this must not be a one-size-fits-all strategy, but a flexible system that welcomes difference and a multiplicity of approaches to supporting people who have dementia. The distinct needs of Indigenous seniors must not be automatically assimilated into dominant crisis-focused discourses and related policy and practice developments. Future research must find ways to listen to the voices and ideas of families like Joe's. Settler populations must acknowledge ongoing colonialism and push their communities and political leaders to generously support reparation – with their hearts and minds, as well as resources, recognition, and respect. This includes actively supporting Indigenous-led visions and approaches to care for Indigenous seniors in their communities.

Acknowledgment

I would like to extend my sincere gratitude to Dr. Susan Strega for her feedback on an early version of this chapter and for her encouragement along the way.

References

Alfred, Taiaiake. 1999. *Peace, Power, Righteousness: An Indigenous Manifesto.* Oxford: Oxford University Press.

Anderson, Mark C., and Carmen Robertson. 2011. *Seeing Red: A History of Natives in Canadian Newspapers.* Winnipeg: University of Manitoba Press.

Bartlett, Ruth, and Deborah O'Connor. 2010. *Broadening the Dementia Debate: Towards Social Citizenship.* Bristol: Policy Press.

Beatty, Belulah B., and Loleen Berdahl. 2011. "Health Care and Aboriginal Seniors in Urban Canada: Helping a Neglected Class." *International Indigenous Policy Journal* 2 (1): 1–16. DOI:10.18584/iipj.2011.2.1.10.

Bracken, Denis C., Lawrence Deane, and Larry Morrissette. 2009. "Desistance and Social Marginalization: The Case of Canadian Aboriginal Offenders." *Theoretical Criminology* 13 (61): 61–78. DOI:10.1177/1362480608100173.

Carabine, Jean. 2001. "Unmarried Motherhood 1830–1990: A Genealogical Analysis." In *Discourse as Data: A Guide for Analysis,* ed. Margaret Wetherell, Stephanie Taylor, and Simeon J. Yates, 267–310. London: Sage.

CBC News. 2012. "Winnipeg Remand Centre Well over Capacity." *CBC News Manitoba,*

February 7. http://www.cbc.ca/news/canada/manitoba/winnipeg-remand-centre-well-over-capacity-1.1224048.

Cheek, Julianne. 2000. *Postmodern and Poststructural Approaches to Nursing Research.* Thousand Oaks: Sage.

Chrisjohn, Roland, and Sherri Young. 2006. *The Circle Game: Shadows and Substance in the Indian Residential School Experience in Canada.* Penticton: Theytus Books. Originally published 1997.

Cohen-Mansfield, Jiska, Marcia S. Marx, Maha Dakheel-Ali, Natalie G. Regier, Khin Thein, and Laurence Freedman. 2010. "Can Agitated Behavior of Nursing Home Residents with Dementia Be Prevented with the Use of Standardized Stimuli?" *Journal of the American Geriatrics Society* 58 (8): 1459–64.

Comack, Elizabeth, and Evan Bowness. 2010. "Dealing the Race Card: Public Discourse on the Policing of Winnipeg's Inner-City Communities." *Canadian Journal of Urban Research* 19 (1): 34–50.

Czyzewski, Karina. 2011. "Colonialism as a Broader Social Determinant of Health." *International Indigenous Policy Journal* 2 (1): 1–10. http://ir.lib.uwo.ca/cgi/viewcontent.cgi?article=1016&context=iipj.

Etowa, Josephine, Charlotte Jesty, and Adele Vukic. 2011. "Indigenous Nurses' Stories: Perspectives on the Cultural Context of Aboriginal Health Care Work." *Canadian Journal of Native Studies* 31 (2): 29–46.

Fiske, Jo-Anne, and Annette J. Browne. 2006. "Aboriginal Citizen, Discredited Medical Subject: Paradoxical Constructions of Aboriginal Women's Subjectivity in Canadian Health Care Policies." *Policy Sciences* 39 (1): 91–111. DOI:10.1007/s11077-006-9013-8.

Foucault, Michel. 1980. *Power/Knowledge: Selected Interviews and Other Writings, 1972–1977,* ed. Colin Gordon; trans. Colin Gordon, Leo Marshall, John Mepham, and Kate Soper. New York: Pantheon Books.

–. 2011. *The Archaeology of Knowledge,* trans. A.M. Sheridan Smith. London: Routledge, Taylor and Francis Group. Originally published 1969.

Furniss, Elizabeth. 2001. "Aboriginal Justice, the Media, and the Symbolic Management of Aboriginal/Euro-Canadian Relations." *American Indian Culture and Research Journal* 25 (2): 1–36.

Gebhard, Amanda. 2012. "Pipeline to Prison: How Schools Shape a Future of Incarceration for Indigenous Youth." *Briarpatch Magazine,* September-October.

Gee, Ellen M., and Gloria M. Gutman, eds. 2000. *The Overselling of Population Aging: Apocalyptic Demography, Intergenerational Challenges, and Social Policy.* Don Mills: Oxford University Press.

Gurney, Matt. 2011a. "The Coming Alzheimer's Crisis." *Toronto National Post,* January 31, A12.

–. 2011b. "Old, Sick ... and Dangerous." *Toronto National Post,* July 29. https://www.pressreader.com/canada/national-post-latest-edition/20110729/283420598300487.

–. 2011c. "Winnipeg Health System Struggling to Deal with Alzheimer's Patient." *Toronto National Post,* March 28. http://news.nationalpost.com/full-comment/matt-gurney

-winnipeg-health-system-struggling-to-deal-with-alzheimers-patient.

Habjan, Sonja, Holly Prince, and Mary Lou Kelley. 2012. "Caregiving for Elders in First Nations Communities: Social System Perspectives on Barriers and Challenges." *Canadian Journal on Aging* 31 (2): 209–22. DOI:10.1017/S071498081200013X.

Harding, Robert. 2006. "Historical Representations of Aboriginal People in the Canadian News Media." *Discourse and Society* 17 (2): 205–35. DOI:10.1177/0957926506058059.

Henry, Frances, and Carol Tator. 2002. *Discourses of Domination: Racial Bias in the Canadian English-Language Press.* Toronto: University of Toronto Press.

Hulko, Wendy, Evelyn Camille, Elisabeth Antifeau, Mike Arnouse, Nicole Bachynski, and Denise Taylor. 2010. "Views of First Nation Elders on Memory Loss and Memory Care in Later Life." *Journal of Cross-Cultural Gerontology* 25 (4): 317–42. DOI:10.1007/s10823-010-9123-9.

Kelly, Miranda D. 2011. "Toward a New Era of Policy: Health Care Service Delivery to First Nations." *International Indigenous Policy Journal* 2 (1): 1–12. http://ir.lib.uwo.ca/cgi/viewcontent.cgi?article=1017&context=iipj.

Kirmayer, Laurence J., Gregory M. Brass, and Caroline L. Tait. 2001. "The Mental Health of Aboriginal Peoples: Transformations of Identity and Community." In *The Mental Health of Indigenous Peoples: Culture and Mental Health Research Unit Report No. 10,* ed. Laurence J. Kirmayer, Mary Ellen Macdonald, and Gregory M. Brass, 5–25. https://www.mcgill.ca/tcpsych/files/tcpsych/Report10.pdf.

Koopman, Colin. 2013. *Genealogy as Critique: Foucault and the Problems of Modernity.* Bloomington: Indiana University Press.

Kovach, Margaret. 2005. "Emerging from the Margins: Indigenous Methodologies." In *Research as Resistance,* ed. Leslie Brown and Susan Strega, 19–36. Toronto: Canadian Scholars' Press.

Kusch, Larry. 2010a. "Aid Comes for Alzheimer's Sufferer." *Winnipeg Free Press,* October 8. http://www.winnipegfreepress.com/local/aid-comes-for-alzheimers-sufferer-104555639.html.

–. 2010b. "Alzheimer's Sufferer Sits in Remand." *Winnipeg Free Press,* October 7. http://www.winnipegfreepress.com/local/alzheimers-sufferer-sits-in-remand-104473169.html.

–. 2010c. "Crown Stays Assault Charge against Alzheimer's Sufferer." *Winnipeg Free Press,* November 3. http://www.winnipegfreepress.com/local/crown-stays-assault-charge-against-alzheimers-sufferer-106596133.html.

–. 2010d. "Dementia Sufferer Released from Jail." *Winnipeg Free Press,* October 9. http://www.winnipegfreepress.com/local/dementia-sufferer-released-from-jail-104625449.html.

–. 2010e. "Family Wants Man with Alzheimer's Moved Out of Remand Centre." *Winnipeg Free Press,* October 6. https://www.winnipegfreepress.com/breakingnews/Family-wants-man-with--104423844.html.

Lanting, Shawnda, Margaret Crossley, Debra Morgan, and Allison Cammer. 2011. "Aboriginal Experiences of Aging and Dementia in a Context of Sociocultural

Change: Qualitative Analysis of Key Informant Group Interviews with Aboriginal Seniors." *Journal of Cross-Cultural Gerontology* 26 (1): 103–17. DOI:10.1007/s10823-010-9136-4.

Lavoie, Josée G. 2004. "The Value and Challenges of Separate Services: First Nations in Canada." In *Accessing Health Care: Responding to Diversity,* ed. Judith Healy and Martin McKee, 325–49. Oxford: Oxford University Press.

Lavoie, Josée G., Evelyn L. Forget, and Annette J. Browne. 2010. "Caught at the Crossroad: First Nations, Health Care, and the Legacy of the Indian Act." *Pimatisiwin: A Journal of Aboriginal and Indigenous Community Health* 8 (1): 83–100.

"Local Alzheimer's Patient Charged in Killing Granted Bail." 2011. *Winnipeg Free Press,* May 28. http://www.winnipegfreepress.com/local/local-alzheimers-patient-charged-in-killing-granted-bail-122766019.html.

"Long-Term Strategy on Aging Required." 2011. *Winnipeg Free Press,* April 6. http://www.winnipegfreepress.com/our-communities/editorial/Long-term-strategy-on-aging-required-119283759.html.

Martin, Melissa. 2011a. "Caring for Reserves' Seniors." *Winnipeg Free Press,* April 2. https://www.winnipegfreepress.com/local/caring-for-reserves-seniors-119110829.html.

–. 2011b. "Family's Anger over Dad's Death Directed at System, Not Accused." *Winnipeg Free Press,* April 1. http://www.winnipegfreepress.com/local/familys-anger-over-dads-death-directed-at-system-not-accused-119048099.html.

McIntyre, Mike. 2012. "Alzheimer's Patient Spared from Trial." *Winnipeg Free Press,* February 25. http://www.winnipegfreepress.com/local/alzheimers-patient-spared-from-trial-140406993.html.

Mitchell, Catherine. 2010. "A Holding Cell as a Proxy for Health Care." *Winnipeg Free Press,* October 9. http://www.winnipegfreepress.com/opinion/analysis/a-holding-cell-as-a-proxy-for-health-care-104625339.html.

O'Connor, Joe. 2011. "Alzheimer's and a Senseless Death in Winnipeg." *Toronto National Post,* March 31. http://news.nationalpost.com/full-comment/joe-oconnor-alzheimers-and-a-senseless-death-in-winnipeg.

"Our Alzheimer's Crisis, in Tragic Microcosm." 2013. *Toronto National Post,* January 7. http://news.nationalpost.com/full-comment/national-post-editorial-board-our-alzheimers-crisis-in-tragic-microcosm.

"Our Growing Elder-Care Crisis." 2013. *Toronto National Post,* March 16. http://news.nationalpost.com/full-comment/national-post-editorial-board-our-growing-elder-care-crisis.

Paul, Alexandra. 2011. "Senior Charged after Assault." *Winnipeg Free Press,* March 27. http://www.winnipegfreepress.com/local/senior-charged-after-assault-118730779.html.

Picard, André. 2010. "We Need a Dementia Strategy, Not Grandpa Prisons." *Toronto Globe and Mail,* October 14.

Robertson, Ann. 1991. "The Politics of Alzheimer's Disease: A Case Study in Apocalyptic

Demography." In *Critical Perspectives on Aging: The Political and Moral Economy of Growing Old*, ed. Meredith Minkler and Carol L. Estes, 135–50. Amityville: Baywood.

Rockwood, Kenneth, and Ron Keren. 2010. "Dementia Services in Canada." *International Journal of Geriatric Psychiatry* 25 (9): 876–80. DOI:10.1002/gps.2590.

Sanders, Carol. 2011. "Probe Death, Family Says." *Winnipeg Free Press*, March 30. http://www.winnipegfreepress.com/local/probe-death-family-says-118898469.html.

Sanders, Carol, and Alexandra Paul. 2011. "Alzheimer's Patient CHARGED." *Winnipeg Free Press*, March 27. http://www.winnipegfreepress.com/local/alzheimers-patient-charged-118730794.html.

Simpson, Leanne. 2008. "Oshkimaadiziig, the New People." In *Lighting the Eighth Fire: The Liberation, Resurgence, and Protection of Indigenous Nations*, ed. Leanne Simpson, 13–21. Winnipeg: Arbeiter Ring.

Smith, Marianne, and Kathleen Buckwalter. 2005. "Behaviours Associated with Dementia." *American Journal of Nursing* 105 (7): 40–53.

Stanner, William Edward Hanley. 1979. *White Man Got No Dreaming: Essays, 1938–1973*. Canberra: Australian National University Press.

Tamboukou, Maria. 1999. "Writing Genealogies: An Exploration of Foucault's Strategies for Doing Research." *Discourse: Studies in the Cultural Politics of Education* 20 (2): 201–17. DOI:10.1080/0159630990200202.

Tuck, Eve, and Michelle Fine. 2007. "Inner Angles: A Range of Ethical Responses to/with Indigenous and Decolonizing Theories." In *Ethical Futures in Qualitative Research: Decolonizing the Politics of Knowledge*, ed. Norman Denzin and Michael Giardina, 145–68. Walnut Creek: Left Coast Press.

Tuck, Eve, and K. Wayne Yang. 2012. "Decolonization Is Not a Metaphor." *Decolonization: Indigeneity, Education and Society* 1 (1): 1–40. http://decolonization.org/index.php/des/article/view/18630.

Van Herk, Kimberley Anne, Dawn Smith, and Caroline Andrew. 2011. "Identity Matters: Aboriginal Mothers' Experiences of Accessing Health Care." *Contemporary Nurse* 37 (1): 57–68. DOI:10.5172/conu.2011.37.1.057.

"Winnipeg Man with Alzheimer's Won't Stand Trial for Manslaughter in Fatal Push." 2012. *Canadian Free Press*, February 24.

COYOTE
Keeper of Memories

Danielle Wilson, Gwen Campbell-McArthur,
Wendy Hulko, Star Mahara, Jean William,
Cecilia DeRose, and Estella Patrick Moller

>> Coyote was sitting atop of Mount Paul one day. He was asking the Sun for help with his children. He had many children and they were always making so many demands on him, day and night. Coyote was very tired. He asked, "Sun, I am tired because of all my children. They are endless in their demands on how to catch fish, to show them how to make pit houses, how to make the fire. Can you help me?"

Sun is quiet for a few minutes and says, "Coyote, you have not helped your children to be self-sufficient. You are doing everything for your children, and you have to teach them how to feed, house, and care for themselves. After that, you will find your peace. But I must let you know ..."

Coyote is very impatient with Sun – she is old and talks slow and pauses often between words. So Coyote listens as long as he can to Sun, and he decides he has heard enough. Coyote interrupts Sun: "Thanks, Sun, that is a great idea and I will do just as you say."

Coyote forgets to be patient and listen to the wisdom of Sun. Coyote is anxious to show his children how to feed, house, and care for themselves. He starts the very next morning. Coyote teaches the men how to gather fish from the rivers, how to hunt deer and rabbit from the forests. He shows the women where to gather berries and asparagus from the earth, how to make clothes for themselves. Coyote shows all his children how to build pit houses and the best places to build them. He teaches his children how to make fire for themselves and how to keep it well.

Coyote is very happy with his teachings. He now has time to sit back and watch his children. But as the sun sets and rises, he is getting bored. He misses the attention from his children. But most troubling is his children are becoming very greedy, they are taking too much berries and fish from Bear, and not enough trees are left for Beaver to use for his home. Sun watches over the days and sees all this happening.

Coyote decides to talk to his children about this. He says to them, "My children, you are not being fair to the other creatures. You are taking everything for yourselves, and others are suffering because you are taking too much yourselves. Bear and Beaver are hungry and cold. They need some fish and trees for themselves too."

The children listen to Coyote and they don't think they are being unfair. They feel that Coyote's teachings are enough to lead them down their own paths and that they are wise enough to manage all that they have learned. They say to Coyote that they don't want to share the food and trees with others. They are afraid that they will not have enough for themselves.

Coyote is stuck, he doesn't know what to do. He decides he needs to talk to Sun again. Maybe Sun has more to tell him. So Coyote climbs up Mount Paul to talk to Sun. He says to Sun, "I don't know what to do. My children are thriving from my teachings, but they are taking too much for themselves, so much that other creatures are suffering because of their greediness. What can I do?"

Sun was waiting for impatient Coyote to come back to her. Sun slowly says, "Coyote, you only listened to half of what I was going to say. Teach your children to thank the Creator before they take what they need, to take only what they need, and to return those parts back to the Creator. Your teachings must be balanced with the giving and taking, Coyote."

Coyote now understands his mistake and wishes he had remembered to be more patient with Sun the first time he talked to her. Coyote knows that his children are very greedy and don't want to share the food and trees. Coyote knows what he needs to do now.

So Coyote says to his children, "My children, you make me so proud – I have taught you well and you are thriving. You have fish and berries for many feasts. Even in the cold winter months, you will be well fed. Your homes are sturdy and warm from the fires. You never go hungry or cold. You have learned very well."

Coyote's children feel their chests swell from the compliments from Coyote. Coyote continued: "But my children, you are not doing as good as Eagle. I taught Eagle to build his own nest and catch his own food all by himself. He doesn't have to share with brother or sister Eagle. Everything he catches, he keeps it to himself and his nest is never crowded. Do you want to learn how to be like Eagle?"

The children talk among themselves. How much easier that each child would like to keep all the fish and berries that they catch and gather to stock for their own use? And to have a pit house all for one person? The children want to learn the Eagle's way because Coyote's children are greedy and want more, and they want to do better than Eagle. Coyote says to them, "For me to teach you Eagle's ways, you must give back my teachings. I will put those teachings in this grass basket and keep them here beside me. When you give back my teachings, I will give you Eagle's teachings so that you won't have to share anything with your brothers and sisters."

Coyote's children are eager for Eagle's teachings, and they forget that Coyote can be a trickster and speaks only half truths. They give their teachings back to Coyote. Coyote says, "I need to teach you about giving and taking, my children. You have taken too much and not given back enough. You are not sharing what you catch and build with your own brothers and sisters. Bear and Beaver are going hungry and have no shelters for themselves. You are not eagles. I am going to keep my teachings in this basket. I will let you use what I think you need. No longer will I let you use all my teachings for yourselves. I will watch over each of you and take back the teachings that I need."

Coyote's children were tricked to give back their teachings. Coyote places the memories in his grass basket beside him. He feels proud of himself for restoring the balance again.

But Coyote forgot about the precious balance of memories in his children. His children now forget too many things, they forget where their pit houses are, brothers and sisters forget each other. Coyote needs to help them with all their daily chores again, and he is getting exhausted again. It is like his children have come full circle to infants. Exhausted, Coyote climbs back up Mount Paul to speak to Sun again. "Sun, please help me. I listened patiently to you last time and heard all that you said, but my children are not any better. They are worse than before and I am so tired. What have I done? How can I change things to be better?"

Sun nourishes the berries and trees, wakes up Bear from hibernation, and warms the land. She is life giving and wants Coyote and his children to survive. So she says, "Coyote, listen to me well. In taking back your teachings, you took back too many memories by accident. Coyote, you did not realize that other memories are attached to your teachings. Memories are all connected, like the grass weaved in a grass basket. You can't pull one piece of grass out without affecting the other grass threads. You have to be careful in what memories you take back."

Again, Coyote sees his mistake – in taking away the traditional teachings of Sun and Eagle, he took away memories important for survival of his children. Coyote needs to remember the sacred teachings and the precious balance of all living things. Coyote needs to be mindful of his own memories basket.

So Coyote reaches into his grass basket and gives back his teachings to his children. And he watches closely over his children to make sure they only take their share of food and trees. When his children start to become forgetful, they know it is because of Coyote and his grass basket. His children understand that Coyote controls the basket of memories and takes them back when he wants to and from whom he wants. Sometimes he keeps the memories for a short time, other times he keeps the memories for a long time. It all depends on how full his grass basket is at the time.

PART 2

INDIGENOUS PERSPECTIVES ON CARE AND PREVENTION

CHAPTER 4

PERCEPTIONS OF DEMENTIA PREVENTION
among Anishinaabe Living on Manitoulin Island

Jessica E. Pace, Kristen Jacklin, Wayne Warry,
and Karen Pitawanakwat

IN 2007, INDIGENOUS COMMUNITIES in Ontario identified Alzheimer's disease and related dementias (ADRD) as a research priority.[1] A roundtable forum documented the perception that ADRD was a growing concern and identified a need for culturally appropriate services and supports related to dementia. Consequently, a provincial research program was developed in collaboration with Manitoulin Island First Nations, which later engaged multiple Indigenous communities in Ontario. This program includes a large ethnographic study titled "Cultural Understandings of Alzheimer's Disease and Related Dementias in Aboriginal Peoples in Ontario", conducted by Kristen Jacklin and Wayne Warry. As part of this larger study, the findings in this chapter represent research with the Wikwemikong Unceded Indian Reserve and member communities of the United Chiefs and Councils of Mnidoo Mnising (UCCMM) on Manitoulin Island, Ontario.

This chapter presents findings specific to Manitoulin Island Anishinaabe understandings of how to prevent dementia and maintain a healthy mind while aging. These understandings are central to our thesis that effective programming for dementia prevention must be culturally grounded and must consider the unique social determinants of health that affect Indigenous people. Our analysis highlights synergies between Indigenous knowledge regarding brain health and dementia and explanations of risk factors for dementia and risk reduction strategies reported in the biomedical literature. In doing so, it elucidates key considerations and approaches to dementia prevention and health promotion strategies for Anishinaabe on Manitoulin Island.

Dementia in Indigenous Populations

Biomedical research has identified several risk factors and prevention strategies concerning dementia. The Alzheimer Society of Canada describes two categories of risk factors: modifiable, which may be influenced by the behaviours or life circumstances of individuals, and non-modifiable, which cannot be changed. The primary non-modifiable risk factors for dementia are age and genetics (Alzheimer Society of Canada 2010). Other conditions, including type 2 diabetes, head injury, stroke, high cholesterol, high blood pressure, mild cognitive impairment, chronic inflammatory conditions, a history of clinical depression, lack of cognitive stimulation, and obesity, also increase dementia risk (Alzheimer Society of Canada 2010). The same is true for a lack of formal/Western education, low socioeconomic status, stress, smoking, and alcohol abuse (Alzheimer Society of Canada 2010). All of these are known risk factors for the mainstream population; however, like prevention, risk may be experienced differently in an Indigenous context.

Recent research shows that dementia rates are rising among First Nations people. Kristen Jacklin, Jennifer Walker, and Marjorie Shawande (2013) suggest that dementia may be more prevalent among Alberta First Nations than among their non–First Nations counterparts. Their research estimates that the age-standardized prevalence of dementia among the former is 7.5 per 1,000, which is higher than the rate of 5.6 per 1,000 in the latter. Derived from administrative health data, this information indicates that, between 1998 and 2009, the prevalence of dementia grew more rapidly in the First Nations population than in the mainstream population, disproportionately affecting males and younger seniors. This is some of the first Canadian evidence to suggest that dementia may now be more prevalent in First Nations than in non–First Nations. Research in Australia has also indicated an increased prevalence of dementia in Indigenous populations and a younger age of onset, as compared to non-Indigenous populations (Smith et al. 2008).

Jacklin, Walker, and Shawande (2013) connect the high prevalence of dementia in Alberta First Nations with a specific constellation of risk factors, which is more ubiquitous among First Nations people than among the non-Indigenous population. These include higher rates of smoking and obesity, as well as the associated illnesses of hypertension, stroke, diabetes, and heart disease. Further, the authors argue that Indigenous people's risk for dementia is shaped by their high vulnerability to the impacts of social determinants of health, including poverty and lower levels of formal education, and potentially by increased rates of post-traumatic stress disorder caused by residential school trauma. Other research also shows differential dementia risks for Indigenous people, including increased susceptibility to vascular dementias because of higher rates of diabetes, cardiovascular disease, and alcoholism (Hendrie et al. 1993). Many of these risks stem from the history of Indigenous peoples, who were marginalized, disenfranchised, and oppressed as a result of colonialism and government interventions (Kirmayer, Simpson, and Cargo 2003). Research concerning Indigenous understandings of dementia further shows that Indigenous people perceive changes in traditional lifeways as contributing to the higher prevalence of dementia (Hulko et al. 2010; Lanting et al. 2011; Pace 2013).

The distinction between biomedical and Indigenous ways of knowing and understanding dementia is relevant to this discussion. Indigenous understandings of health and being well are holistic and less deterministic than biomedicine, which considers aging to be a state of biologically based functional decline and sees dementia as a pathology. By contrast, it has been documented that Indigenous peoples tend to perceive age-associated memory loss and confusion as normal, natural, and accepted (Cammer 2006; Henderson and Henderson 2002; Hulko et al. 2010; Jacklin and Warry 2012; Lanting et al. 2011). The development of childlike traits and the return of old memories are seen as expected parts of aging (Sutherland 2007). However, the perception that dementia is a "terrible disease" (Hulko et al. 2010, 328), frightening, or worrisome (Pace 2013) has also been documented in Indigenous settings, particularly for the later stages of the condition. This reflects a tension between Indigenous and biomedical understandings of dementia. Such cultural perceptions potentially play a significant role in shaping preventive behaviours and early diagnosis and intervention, as Indigenous individuals may not perceive mild symptoms as pathological and may resist using Western medicines to address confusion and memory loss (Pace 2013).

Healthy diet, aerobic exercise, cognitive stimulation, and an active social life are all thought to help prevent the onset of dementia in the general population (Alzheimer Society of Canada 2010; Larson et al. 2006; Middleton and Yaffe 2009). Limiting alcohol consumption, smoking, and stress, preventing head injury, managing vascular risk factors, and seeking treatment for medical conditions such as diabetes and high blood pressure can also aid in the maintenance of brain health (Alzheimer Society of Canada 2010; Middleton and Yaffe 2009).

Understandings of Anishinaabe people's risk for dementia and their ability to engage in preventive behaviours must reflect on social and Indigenous determinants of health (Reading and Wein 2009). Mainstream dementia prevention resources do not consider the unique social, political, and historical context in which Indigenous people live. This is significant because although individuals can control their behaviour, they can do so only within the limits determined by their environment, personal circumstances, and life history. For this reason, we need to be cautious when referring to mainstream concepts such as "modifiable" risk factors, which infers control and choice over one's circumstances and does not adequately reflect the lived reality of marginalized groups, let alone those who remain under colonial structures and policies. The idea that a risk is modifiable must be carefully articulated and considered to avoid placing blame on the individual for failing to engage in risk-reduction behaviours. To do this, we need a framework that addresses the larger social and structural barriers that inhibit individuals from changing their health behaviours, even if they are aware of the potential benefits of doing so.

The failure to attend to social determinants of health in mainstream approaches to prevention aimed at Indigenous people suggests a lack of cultural safety (Brascoupé and Waters 2009), which can hinder Indigenous individuals from relating to dementia prevention advice. Cultural safety, a concept originally defined by Māori nurse educators in New Zealand, addresses structural inequalities and power relationships between health care providers and patients (Ramsden 1990). The Aboriginal Nurses Association of Canada describes cultural safety as moving beyond cultural sensitivity (respecting difference) and cultural competence (gaining skills, knowledge, and attitudes). Instead, many frameworks for cultural safety attend to structural inequalities in the system of health care delivery (ANAC 2009).

Although no previous research has focused specifically on Indigenous understandings of dementia prevention, some studies have considered culturally appropriate prevention strategies for health issues such as diabetes, heart disease, and mental illness in Indigenous communities. Some of these works highlight the importance of political empowerment, culturally grounded community healing, and strengthening ethnocultural identity and community integration as key to enhancing health (Chandler and Lalonde 1998; Jacklin and Warry 2012; Kirmayer, Simpson, and Cargo 2003; Warry 1998).

Research Site

Our research was carried out in seven First Nations communities on Manitoulin Island, which lies near the north shore of Lake Huron, in northern Ontario. These communities (Wikwemikong, Sheshegwaning, M'Chigeeng, Zhibaahaasing, Sheguiandah, Aundeck Omni Kaning, and Whitefish River) range in size from seventy-six to three thousand residents. The Indigenous population of Manitoulin is primarily Ojibwe, Odawa, and Potawatomi. Manitoulin was selected in part because of the diversity of the seven First Nations in size, remoteness, and access to services. In addition, key stakeholders at the community level had expressed an interest in engaging in research about dementia.

Research Approach

As mentioned earlier, the data presented in this chapter are drawn from a multi-sited ethnographic study. Its purpose was to gather foundational information about knowledge, attitudes, beliefs, and behaviours relating to ADRD in diverse Indigenous communities in Ontario. To gather data, we used qualitative ethnographic methods, including participant observation, semi-structured interviews, key informant interviews, and focus groups with health care providers. This chapter reports on a subset of data that are specific to dementia prevention in Indigenous communities. A community-based researcher (Karen Pitawanakwat) and a PhD student (Jessica Pace) conducted in-depth interviews with seniors (aged fifty-five or older), people with dementia, and traditional knowledge keepers (Table 4.1). Participants were selected using convenience sampling. Informants from Manitoulin UCCMM communities were identified by the researcher (Pace), with assistance from the home care nurse manager from Mnaamodzawin Health Services. Participants in Wikwemikong were identified by Pitawanakwat, who is also a nurse at the local health centre. These community health workers asked potential interviewees if they were interested in being contacted by a researcher about being involved in the study.

Participants were asked how people in their community could prevent dementia and keep a healthy mind as they aged. Interview questions aimed to identify the barriers and enablers to prevention, including personal and structural factors that might influence a person's ability to engage in preventive behaviours or reap the benefits of protective factors.

TABLE 4.1 Interview participants

Research site	Wikwemikong (W)	UCCMM communities (M)	Total
Interviews			
People with dementia	5	5	10
Seniors (≥ age 55)	6	4	10
Traditional knowledge keepers		2	2
Total	11	11	22

NOTE: A local advisory group for the project directed the team to use "senior" to describe research participants who were fifty-five or older. The word "Elder" is reserved for those who hold special status in the community, so the researchers avoided it. However, interviewees often used "elder" and "senior" interchangeably.

A critical interpretive theoretical framework (Scheper-Hughes 1990) and a post-colonial lens, in consultation with community stakeholders, guided data analysis. This approach recognizes inequalities in health care and services to marginalized groups and understands health issues in the context of broader political and economic forces (Baer, Singer, and Susser 2003). We used phenomenological thematic analysis to identify themes in the interview data that were related to causes and prevention of dementia. Indigenous experiences and conceptualizations related to prevention were isolated and compared against known biomedical risk factors and risk reduction strategies to identify similarities and differences. Anishinaabe understandings of prevention were further considered by the Anishinaabe author (Pitawanakwat), with the assistance of a community advisory group.

Perspectives of Dementia among Manitoulin Island Anishinaabe

Our analysis revealed that several participants connected prevention with finding balance between the quadrants of the Anishinaabe medicine wheel over the life course. This view was held by individuals in every participant group (people with dementia, seniors, and traditional knowledge keepers). There were no substantial differences in the perceptions of each group. To respect these Anishinaabe interpretations, we organized our data in relation to four major themes concerning prevention: physical, mental, emotional, and spiritual. Much like the Anishinaabe medicine wheel, our analysis demonstrates the interconnectedness of the quadrants and the importance of balance when discussing prevention. Our intention is to demonstrate how people perceive the interrelatedness among ethnocultural identity, practices, language, and cognition to begin to think about how Indigenous knowledge may guide dementia prevention strategies targeted to this population.

Physical Quadrant

Because participants believed that healthy lifestyle behaviours protected against cognitive decline, the physical quadrant is involved in dementia prevention. Minimizing risks such as head injury and exposure to contaminants was also seen as important.

Consuming fresh and healthy foods, particularly those that could be harvested or hunted, was emphasized as a component of maintaining brain health. One senior remarked,

> My grandmother or grandfather didn't have [dementia], but they were very old. I don't know why they didn't get it, but maybe it is the way we eat, too. I'll talk about it again here; they always planted food, had gardens and preserved what was full grown. They got everything they needed to live, they had farm animals, chickens, everything was there. You didn't go anywhere to buy anything you had. So this might be where it comes from because now everything is sold, what people are selling, companies, no one knows what is done to the food that is cooked. Vegetables, everything, there is too much of what is going to ruin you as a living person. (senior02W)[2]

Herbs and traditional medicines were perceived as important dietary supplements that had protective benefits. Participants described that "food is medicine, and medicine is food" as an example of the importance of "eating fresh." Eating fresh was seen as protective because traditional food procurement activities such as hunting and gardening require physical and mental exertion, with the additional benefit of producing healthy foods that seniors can eat. Hunting, for example, relies on skills that draw on several cognitive processes, including dreaming, planning, memory, and knowledge of the land. Discussing seniors who hunted, fished, and gardened, a traditional knowledge keeper said,

A lot of them are, still very active doing those [cultural activities]. The elderly population we see are the ones that are actually very active in doing those things, so they're doing it and their brains are very good because they're doing those things. Those ones we don't see are the ones that are actually more into being diagnosed with Alzheimer's because they're not engaging in that. They're eating stuff that's bought in the store and with all the additives in it, and the people we see that are in the traditional healing program are the ones that are engaging in those things – they go hunting, they go fishing, and they have little gardens. So they're growing their own food and cooking for themselves and doing all those activities [as] part of their self-care. (traditional01M)

Food additives and environmental contaminants were a significant concern and were believed to cause illness. This link between sickness and the environment has also been documented in other Indigenous contexts (Cassady 2007; Tyrell 2007). A senior noted, "Actually it's funny how we're living because this, this whole earth is contaminated. Everything you eat now is no good. That's why a lot of people are sick. This whole earth is contaminated" (senior05M).

Participants believed that avoiding contaminants was an essential part of maintaining a healthy brain. However, they described a tension between their desire to eat wild foods and their understanding that these were less healthy than they had been in the past. Ingesting contaminants was linked to the development of toxins in the blood that were perceived to harm the brain. Prescription medicines were understood to have similar effects:

We're always taking some kind of pill, you know? Blood pressure pill, sugar diabetes pill, that's why you, that's why you get that 'cause your liver, your liver is full of toxins and your, your blood is not right. That's why you get all that. Your blood just plugs up the brain, so your brain cells die out because of the, you know, the plugging of the brain with all those [pills]. (senior05M)

Several participants said that avoiding prescription drugs was important to maintaining a healthy mind. This was seen as a challenge, as many felt that doctors frequently over-prescribed medication.

In a related vein, abstaining from alcohol consumption, smoking, and substance abuse was seen as helping to prevent cognitive problems:

> Alcohol and there's even the way we eat, too, that's been mentioned too. Smoking, people that smoke. 'Cause, you know, when you drink, you're actually kind of taking something from your, you know, you forget and you forget and you kind of well, especially if you get drunk so, in the long run you're actually doing something to your health, your brain. (senior03M)

Participants were especially vocal about the impacts of alcohol and referred to the immediate and long-term effects of drinking on cognitive function. Alcohol and substance abuse were understood to impede individuals from engaging in mental stimulation through avenues such as oral history, ritual, and other cultural practices.

Finally, interviewees recognized a link between head trauma and dementia. They explained that some head injuries immediately impaired cognitive function and that those sustained during childhood could cause memory problems later in life. Some participants felt that avoiding situations in which they might hit their head could aid in preventing dementia.

Mental Quadrant

Participants recognized the importance of cognitive stimulation and described specific activities to exercise the brain. Thus, the mental quadrant is relevant to dementia prevention.

Cognitive stimulation emerged as the most effective method of averting dementia. Participants mentioned word and number games, reading, and playing cards, Bingo, and computer games as key to deterring memory loss. These activities, which often involved beneficial social interaction, were understood to exercise the brain, requiring the use of memory, problem-solving skills, and quick thinking:

> You constantly have to exercise that part of the brain to keep it active, instead of just stagnating and just sitting there and just watching TV where you're not actually thinking and engaging in something new,

eh? You're watching other people live, versus being active in it, eh? ...
I visualize the brain as a muscle that if you don't use it, then it's, you're
going to end up with dementia because you're not using it, so you
have to put new information in there all the time to keep it active.
(traditionalo1M)

Learning new skills was also seen as beneficial. However, formal Western
education was not necessarily identified as an important source of cognitive
stimulation. Experiential knowledge and the ability to share knowledge
through storytelling and teaching were more highly valued. Storytelling and
teaching engaged cognitive processes such as planning and short- and long-
term memory. They also promoted emotional engagement and social contact,
and they fostered intergenerational relationships, reinforcing traditional
family and community roles.

Other sources of cognitive stimulation included keeping a calendar,
writing reminders, cooking, crafting, sewing, meditation, and art therapy.
Crafting, in particular, was seen as an important source of complex cognitive
stimulation. In addition, engaging with Anishinaabe culture through ceremony, language, and traditional roles in family and community was seen
to play a multifaceted part in stimulating the brain.

Emotional Quadrant

The emotional quadrant emerged as crucial to dementia prevention because
in the Anishinaabe worldview, feelings and emotion are inextricable from
thought. Thus, healing from trauma and avoiding stress were important.
Relationships and social stimulation were believed to protect against depression, loneliness, and isolation, which were understood to increase dementia risk.

Poor health, stress, grief related to deaths in a family or community,
problems with community youth, job loss, historical trauma, and residential
school experiences were described as detrimental to cognitive health:

The things that we have seen and I've heard about also is that any
trauma, any type of trauma can, effects the holism of the individual,
which is, the brain is related to that part, the emotions, the physical,
and the spiritual. So, when somebody is traumatized, you know, it is
all those areas that are affected. So, if you don't get that healing for
those areas, that is one of the first areas you'll see is the brain, the effect

on the brain. People will disassociate themselves, so that imbalance also affects the brain, because of the trauma. They're never the same again. So, unless you do the healing for that, because a lot of our people have shifted away from traditional healing, and mainstream therapy has a different approach, you know, a lot of times for any kind of trauma you are medicated. So, and then the medication actually affects the brain too, so the person can be heavily medicated, and they won't be moving around or they won't be doing anything because they're depressed so they, but it's actually the chances of healing from that trauma is questionable. (traditional01M)

Since stress and trauma cannot always be avoided, healing from trauma was thought to prevent problems with brain health.

Social contact, including visiting or talking on the phone, was seen as beneficial for emotional health. Intergenerational social contact, especially with children, was perceived as an opportunity for seniors to be made useful and to share their knowledge. This relationship has been disrupted in many communities, and efforts to re-establish links between seniors and youth were thought to contribute to social and cognitive stimulation, which would benefit the well-being of seniors:

> They should be made useful in sharing their knowledge, make them feeling useful, eh? But it doesn't happen. They'd be very proud to think that they are useful. I thought of doing that, I used to start the long-term-care program ... and that's what I was thinking about doing, bringing in the elders and the kindergarten kids together so they can exchange or talk to each other, or visit the nursing home, those young kids from the kindergarten. (traditional02M)

Human relationships were perceived to help ward off isolation, loneliness, and depression. Seniors who had strong relationships tended to be involved in oral history, visiting, talking, and teaching, which promote self-worth. Having a purpose and engaging in positive interactions with family and youth were described as important contributors to keeping the mind healthy.

Participants suggested that changes to housing and family structures made it more difficult for seniors to access adequate social stimulation than in the past. Extended families that lived together were a key component of traditional lifestyles, which provided seniors with regular access to social stimulation and prevented isolation:

> I think it's something that gets to be the way it is because of, say, family loss, stress, depression, financial [constraints]. I guess the other thing is all your children are living in their own homes. There is no one left to visit with you. Loneliness, I think. It's not like that any more, the so-called extended family; now it's just linear [sic] families. (senior04W)

Today, it is less common for extended families to reside together, and some families are separated by large geographical distances. Participants suggested that this disrupted family structure and prevented seniors from benefitting from familial support and important roles, including caring for grandchildren, keeping the fire, and engaging in intergenerational contact. Interviewees believed that seniors were less prone to dementia in the past because they had regular access to family and were able to take part in cognitively engaging activities.

Humour, an important mechanism for helping people to maintain a positive outlook and come to terms with emotional difficulties, was also seen as a benefit of social contact. Humour was closely linked to speaking the Anishinaabe language, Anishinaabemowin, which was thought to promote laughter. A traditional knowledge keeper stated that it

> is a fun language, there's a lot of humour attached to it, so it's good for the brain because of that ... You say something in English, people usually don't [laugh] unless they mispronounce the word and then you'll be laughing. We joke a lot, you know ... It's part of our culture, and even if you're forgetting stuff we joke about that too, eh? So it's part of, you know, you joke with somebody, you tease them, eh? "You forgot this," or, "put on the wrong boots," something like that and we laugh about things like that, so people remember when you joke and say, "I'm not doing that again, eh?" So, it's a reminder versus, you know, "somebody's ridiculing me" and feeling bad about it. You can take the joke and it also helps you to remember that you're not going to repeat that. Exactly. So it's, it's good to use the language because it's also part of the long-term memory; they grew up with that language, and then another thing we're doing is also getting them to share their teachings in the language. (traditional01M)

Not only was speaking the language thought to have protective benefits, but the Anishinaabemowin words for "heart" and "feeling" are closely connected to the root word for "mind," indicating how deeply language, emotion, and cognition are intertwined in Anishinaabe life.

Spiritual Quadrant

Spirituality was described as a way of being or living, and a disconnect with spirituality was thought to hinder people from adhering to preventive behaviours, making the spiritual quadrant relevant to the avoidance of dementia. Participants on Manitoulin Island followed various spiritual teachings, but common associations were found. Ceremony and prayer were identified as an important way of engaging with spirituality that also benefitted people as a source of cognitive stimulation:

> I strongly believe in prayer, eh? Every day first thing when I get up, I pray, no matter what. I'm still praying ... and during the day I sit and read the Bible, eh, the Word. And then at the end of the day again, I pray before I go to bed or else if I don't I'd be scared to live alone, but when I pray I know that I'm not alone. (person with dementia03W)

Some participants said that sweat lodge ceremonies allowed people to clear their mind of problems, which promoted cognitive and emotional health:

> We go in a sweat lodge and purify your, try and purify yourself, and you can talk with whatever is troubling you while you're in there. And it stays in there, you don't bring anything out what's said in the sweat lodge ... And when you go in the sweat lodge, when you cleanse yourself, your mind comes clear, eh? You can cry, whatever you want to do. When you come out of there, you've got a clear, clearer head and know what you should be trying to do with yourself to get rid of whatever problem you have. Problems you have are supposed to be taken away when you are in the sweat lodge. (senior04M)

Ceremonies were perceived as beneficial because they were complex and required the memorization of steps, songs, and teachings. When they lead ceremonies, Elders normally rely solely on memory and do not use notes. The content of specific ceremonies was also linked to broader knowledge and memories of other rituals and seasonally based cultural activities. Involvement in ceremonies gave seniors a purpose, provided cognitive stimulation, and connected them with their spirituality:

Well, when we used to have the ceremonies down here, eh, it was the old people who were the leaders and even if, say, I do know how to run this ceremony, but I would still ask that older person, "Is this what I do next?" Even though I know it. So this person says, "Yah, that's what you do, that is the song," so that they feel their importance in there, they are worth something, you think highly of them. Even though you know how to run that ceremony. (senior04W)

Some participants explained the importance of spirituality in relation to teachings of the medicine wheel, focusing on balance between the spiritual, mental, emotional, and physical realms:

Well, it has to do with your, with your mind, and, you know, that's why I tried to share with you, that being able to balance your life and ways that helps you to put your thoughts, your feelings, your actions, and acceptance in that, sort of balanced way so that a lot had to do with, like, this Elder said to me, "You're out of balance," you know? When I first went to him for help, all he said was, "You're out of balance," so I think that Alzheimer's is being out of balance, for me anyways. So that's why I look at it not being able to function in a balanced way to your thoughts, your feelings, and your actions and acceptance. (senior01W)

The Anishinaabe language also reoccurred as a theme in connection with spirituality. The ability to speak it enabled people to engage more fully in other aspects of cultural and community life:

That is very helpful to have your language. Way back then, people had the real closeness to nature and their surroundings, the environment, the animals. There was this spiritual connection, and it was the language that bonded or put these two things together. When you do use your language, there is some connection to that animal or the Creator, more close relationship, and I think also people are, when they use the language, they are more spiritual. So in that way, they are able to talk to their surroundings; if they're in trouble they'll talk to their surroundings, they'll just go isolate themselves and meditate, which gives you a good feeling and a healthy mind. You have to balance all those things together, body, mind, and spirit, and if one is affected, then the other part gets affected, so you have to work on all those areas to make yourself healthy. (traditional02M)

Speaking and praying in Anishinaabemowin were perceived to more deeply connect people to their spirituality, larger cultural structures, and the world around them, than using English did.

Envisioning a Culturally Safe Approach to Dementia Prevention

Our research revealed that the Anishinaabe of Manitoulin Island connect maintaining a healthy mind and preventing dementia with engagement in life and a healthy lifestyle achieved through balancing emotional, physical, spiritual, and mental health. Our analysis clearly shows that no single behaviour or activity was thought to avert dementia; instead, a combination of factors was required, related to cognitive stimulation, culture, spirituality, healing from trauma, and maintaining good health. Relationships and emotional well-being were viewed as inseparable from overall health and the avoidance of dementia in old age. Participants also recognized the value of prevention and interventions early in the life course so that younger generations could benefit.

Interviewees' understandings of dementia prevention relate closely to their holistic views regarding health, which are sometimes associated with the teachings of the medicine wheel. The medicine wheel refers to a worldview and explanatory model that many Indigenous nations use in a variety of ways (Lavallée 2009). It is represented visually by a circle whose four equal quadrants are associated with the four compass points. The quadrants represent the mental, spiritual, physical, and emotional aspects of the self (Rheault 1999), which are understood to be interconnected. Medicine wheel teachings often stress the balance between qualities that are associated with the four directions. Balance is struck at the centre of the wheel, where "self" is represented. Among Manitoulin Island Anishinaabe, health is equated with Minobimaadiziwin (the Way of a Good Life), which is achieved by striving to balance mental, physical, emotional, and spiritual health (Rheault 1999). Minobimaadiziwin encompasses ideas of the life course, where health (way of a good life) is part of one's lifetime journey around the medicine wheel. To achieve Minobimaadiziwin, one must work toward prevention of illnesses by living well mentally, physically, emotionally, and spiritually (Rheault 1999).

This holistic understanding of dementia, its causes, and its deterrence has been documented in other Canadian First Nations. In particular, our results agree with similar data from a study with a British Columbia First Nation in which seniors said that social contact, the maintenance of overall health, and exercising the mind, body, and spirit were key to brain health (Hulko et al. 2010). Social and environmental causes for dementia linked with the impacts of colonialism and changing ways of life have also been documented elsewhere (Hulko et al. 2010; Lanting et al. 2011).

Recommendations for health promotion related to dementia must consider the interconnectedness of these quadrants and how they relate to broader cultural understandings of health and well-being. Dementia prevention programs should concentrate on integrating multiple spheres of prevention (physical, emotional, mental, spiritual) instead of isolating discrete components. For example, targeting individual seniors and recommending that they "get more exercise" is almost meaningless unless that suggestion takes into account cultural understandings and expectations of exercise and potential structural barriers in Indigenous communities (Thompson, Gifford, and Thorpe 2000). A fitness program focused on physical health outcomes will be less effective than one that is based on hunting or living on the land, which integrate all four quadrants of the medicine wheel. Similarly, ceremonial or other cultural activities require complex cognitive functioning and engage the brain in tasks that require memory, planning, and experiential knowledge. Beyond these cognitive elements, these activities draw on physical skills and relate to spirituality and a connectedness to land and culture.

Traditional crafting is a preventive activity that promotes balance by engaging multiple elements across the quadrants of the medicine wheel. When creating regalia and other articles (such as medicine bags), people must draw on their personal identity and spirituality, using their unique name, animal helpers, and colours to inform the design of the beadwork. Crafting entails engagement with faith, healing, prayer, ritual, and ceremony as individuals draw on the spiritual strength of their animal helpers and the colours that represent their connectedness to the world. Further, the beadwork is complex and requires skill and practice. Hunting, which involves physical activity, provides healthy food and necessitates the use of cognitive processes, including memory and experiential knowledge. Planning a hunt similarly relates closely to spirituality and connectedness because it encompasses seasonal knowledge, ritual, and dreaming. Importantly, prevention activities discussed by participants most often involved connections and relationships rather than individualized activities. Relational aspects were sometimes connections to the spirit world or the land, but also to community, community members, and family, with a strong emphasis on intergenerational contact, which has been disrupted by residential schools and the child welfare policies of the recent past.

The impact of the colonial legacy was interlaced throughout the findings, especially in interviewee observations that dementia was a new condition, caused in part by the relinquishment of traditional lifeways, in which people lived in extended family groups, seniors had clearly defined roles, and intergenerational closeness and cultural continuity were greater. Participants' descriptions of their concerns about dementia suggested that as these lifestyle characteristics became disrupted, so too were their protective effects on cognitive health. The point here is that all the factors that mainstream health care providers see as modifiable are heavily influenced by social determinants of health, which affect populations differently and Indigenous populations uniquely. The word "modifiable" infers choice and control, which we have tried to demonstrate has been removed from this population over the course of history.

Implications

If dementia prevention is to be achieved in Indigenous communities, supports must be implemented at multiple levels – policy, community, family, individual – to encourage healthy behaviours. We reiterate here that health promotion activities need to move beyond simply targeting the individual. Instead, programs need to recognize the impacts of social and Indigenous determinants of health and integrate higher-level supports that make it easier for people to engage in appropriate programming. For example, communities need to be made safer so that seniors feel comfortable going out for walks. Additionally, programming that helps Anishinaabe seniors get involved in cultural activities that incorporate medicine wheel teachings needs to be made available on Manitoulin Island. Parallels in Indigenous understandings of dementia that have been documented elsewhere suggest that similar approaches to prevention may be relevant across a broad Indigenous context.

There is a need to support dementia prevention in Indigenous communities by diminishing the risk factors that are unique to them, addressing the impact of the colonial legacy and the loss of traditional ways of living, and stimulating healing from intergenerational trauma. Health promotion processes should be firmly rooted within the values of respect, caring, equity, and self-determination, and community members should have an active role in defining, designing, and implementing programs that reflect their needs, values, and understandings of health (Kirmayer, Simpson, and Cargo 2003). This is crucial, because even well-designed health promotion programming may fail if it is not culturally safe and does not meet the needs of the community to whom it is directed (Steenbeek 2004).

❖❖❖

On the surface, biomedical recommendations for dementia prevention appear to have much in common with the avoidance measures described by our research participants. Both centre on healthy behaviours throughout the life course (diet, exercise, managing overall health) and continued cognitive and social stimulation. However, biomedical recommendations do not resonate with many Anishinaabe people because they do not reflect their understanding of health and well-being. Biomedical approaches and messages fail to recognize the importance of culture in prevention strategies for dementia in Indigenous populations. Nor do they take into account the unique social determinants of Indigenous people's health and the way these determinants influence the capacity of individuals to engage in preventive behaviours. Our analysis shows that if they are to be meaningful, dementia prevention strategies must be created in partnership with Indigenous communities and be tailored to address the unique risk factors that influence the health of Indigenous people. They must focus on incorporating cultural activities that help individuals achieve "whole" health by tending to physical, mental, emotional, spiritual, and relational aspects of the self.

Acknowledgments

Chi Miigwitch to all the individuals and organizations on Manitoulin Island who contributed their time and knowledge to this project. A special thanks to the staff at Mnaamodzawin Health Services, the Noojmowin Teg Health Centre, and the Wikwemikong Health Centre for their support, especially to Debbie Selent for her assistance in recruiting participants. This research was funded by the Alzheimer Society of Canada, the Ontario Mental Health Foundation, and the Canadian Institutes of Health Research Doctoral Award.

Notes

1 Currently, "Indigenous" and "Aboriginal" both refer to the peoples whose ancestors originally inhabited the territory that is now Canada and the United States. The words encompass First Nations, Inuit, and Métis populations. In this chapter, we primarily use the increasingly more accepted "Indigenous" to refer to the first peoples of Canada.

2 The codes that follow each quotation indicate the group of participants from which the passage was drawn: seniors, traditional knowledge keepers, or people with dementia. For example, the code for the quote above indicates that the speaker is senior number 2 from Wikwemikong. An "M" in the code shows that the speaker is from a United Chiefs and Councils of Mnidoo Mnising community.

References

Alzheimer Society of Canada. 2010. "Rising Tide: The Impact of Dementia on Canadian Society." http://alzheimer.ca/sites/default/files/files/chapters-on/york/rising_tide_full_report_eng_final.pdf.

ANAC (Aboriginal Nurses Association of Canada). 2009. *Cultural Competence and Cultural Safety in Nursing Education: A Framework for First Nations, Inuit and Metis Nursing.* Ottawa: ANAC.

Baer, H., M. Singer, and I. Susser. 2003. "Theoretical Perspectives in Medical Anthropology." In H. Baer, M. Singer, and I. Susser, *Medical Anthropology and the World System,* 31–55. Westport, CT: Praeger.

Brascoupé, Simon, and Catherine Waters. 2009. "Cultural Safety: Exploring the Applicability of the Concept of Cultural Safety to Aboriginal Health and Community Wellness." *International Journal of Aboriginal Health* 5 (2): 6–41.

Cammer, Allison Lee. 2006. "Negotiating Culturally Incongruent Healthcare Systems: The Process of Accessing Dementia Care in Northern Saskatchewan." Master's thesis, University of Saskatchewan.

Cassady, J. 2007. "A Tundra of Sickness: The Uneasy Relationship between Toxic Waste, TEK, and Cultural Survival." *Arctic Anthropology* 44: 87–97.

Chandler, Michael J., and Christopher Lalonde. 1998. "Cultural Continuity as a Hedge against Suicide in Canada's First Nations." *Transcultural Psychiatry* 35 (2): 191–219.

Henderson, J. Neil, and L. Carson Henderson. 2002. "Cultural Construction of Disease: A 'Supernormal' Construct of Dementia in an American Indian Tribe." *Journal of Cross-Cultural Gerontology* 17 (3): 197–212.

Hendrie, H.C., et al. 1993. "Alzheimer's Disease Is Rare in Cree." *International Psycho-geriatrics* 5 (1): 5–14.

Hulko, Wendy, Evelyn Camille, Elisabeth Antifeau, Mike Arnouse, Nicole Bachynksi, and Denise Taylor. 2010. "Views of First Nation Elders on Memory Loss and Memory Care in Later Life." *Journal of Cross-Cultural Gerontology* 25 (4): 317–42.

Jacklin, Kristen M., Jennifer D. Walker, and Marjory Shawande. 2013. "The Emergence of Dementia as a Health Concern among First Nations Populations in Alberta, Canada." *Canadian Journal of Public Health* 104 (1): e39–e44.

Jacklin, K., and W. Warry. 2012. "Decolonizing First Nations Health." In *Health in Rural Canada,* ed. Judith C. Kulig and Allison M. Williams, 373–89. Vancouver: UBC Press.

Kirmayer, Laurence, Cori Simpson, and Margaret Cargo. 2003. "Healing Traditions: Culture, Community and Mental Health Promotion with Canadian Aboriginal Peoples." *Australasian Psychiatry* 11 (1): S15–S23. DOI:10.1046/j.1038-5282.2003.02010.x.

Lanting, Shawnda, Margaret Crossley, Debra Morgan, and Allison Cammer. 2011. "Aboriginal Experiences of Aging and Dementia in a Context of Sociocultural Change: Qualitative Analysis of Key Informant Group Interviews with Aboriginal Seniors." *Journal of Cross-Cultural Gerontology* 26 (1): 103–17.

Larson, Eric B., Li Wang, James D. Bowen, Wayne C. McCormick, Linda Teri, Paul Crane, and Walter Kukull. 2006. "Exercise Is Associated with Reduced Risk for Incident Dementia among Persons 65 Years of Age and Older." *Annals of Internal Medicine* 144 (2): 73–81.

Lavallée, Lynn F. 2009. "Practical Application of an Indigenous Research Framework and Two Qualitative Indigenous Research Methods: Sharing Circles and Anishnaabe Symbol-Based Reflection." *International Journal of Qualitiative Methods* 8 (1): 21–40.

Middleton, Laura E., and Kristine Yaffe. 2009. "Promising Strategies for the Prevention of Dementia." *Archives of Neurology* 66: 1210–15.

Pace, Jessica E. 2013. "Meanings of Memory: Understanding Aging and Dementia in First Nations Communities on Manitoulin Island, Ontario." PhD diss., McMaster University.

Ramsden, I. 1990. "Cultural Safety." *New Zealand Nursing Journal. Kai Tiaki* 83: 18–19.

Reading, Charlotte, and Fred Wein. 2009. *Health Inequalities and Social Determinants of Aboriginal Peoples' Health.* Prince George, BC: National Collaborating Centre for Aboriginal Health.

Rheault, D'Arcy. 1999. *Anishinaabe Mono-Bimaadiziwin: The Way of a Good Life.* Peterborough: Debwewin Press.

Scheper-Hughes, Nancy. 1990. "Three Propositions for a Critically Applied Medical Anthropology." *Social Science and Medicine* 30 (2): 189–97.

Smith, K., L. Flicker, N.T. Lautenschlager, O.P. Almeida, D. Atkinson, A. Dwyer, and D. LoGiudice. 2008. "High Prevalence of Dementia and Cognitive Impairment in Indigenous Australians." *Neurology* 71: 1470–73.

Steenbeek, Audrey. 2004. "Empowering Health Promotion: A Holistic Approach in Preventing Sexually Transmitted Infections among First Nations and Inuit

Adolescents in Canada." *Journal of Holistic Nursing* 22 (3): 254–66.

Sutherland, M.E. 2007, March. "Alzheimer's Disease and Related Dementias (ADRD) in Aboriginal Communities: New Visions and Understandings." Paper presented at Alzheimer's Disease and Related Dementias within Aboriginal Individuals – Roundtable Forum, Sudbury, ON.

Thompson, Samantha J., Sandra M. Gifford, and Lisa Thorpe. 2000. "The Social and Cultural Context of Risk and Prevention: Food and Physical Activity in an Urban Aboriginal Community." *Health Education and Behaviour* 27 (6): 725–43.

Tyrell, Martina. 2007. "Making Sense of Contaminants: A Case Study of Arviat, Nunavut." *Arctic* 59: 370–80.

Warry, Wayne. 1998. *Unfinished Dreams: Community Healing and the Reality of Aboriginal Self-Government.* Toronto: University of Toronto Press.

CHAPTER 5

THE UNDERSTANDING FROM WITHIN PROJECT
Perspectives from Indigenous Caregivers

Carrie Bourassa, Melissa Blind, Kristen Jacklin,
Eric Oleson, and Kate Ross-Hopley

HOW DO INDIGENOUS WOMEN, both those living with a neurological condition and their caregivers, conceptualize and experience dementia? This was one of the questions explored in the Understanding from Within Project, a joint research venture of the Native Women's Association of Canada (NWAC); a research team led by Carrie Bourassa, who was based at the time at First Nations University of Canada; and the Public Health Agency of Canada.[1] One of thirteen projects funded through the umbrella of the four-year National Population Health Study of Neurological Conditions (NPHSNC), it alone focused exclusively on Indigenous people.[2] We chose to focus on Indigenous women because they tend to live longer than Indigenous men (Statistics Canada 2011b); they represent the majority of caregivers in their communities (paid and unpaid) (Hennessy and John 1995, 1996; Korn et al. 2009); and their challenges in accessing care differ from those of Indigenous men (First Nations Regional Health Survey n.d.). This does not mean that we excluded Indigenous men from sharing their stories. They were welcome to take part in individual interviews and research circles. Individuals were not required to have an official diagnosis in order to participate. Nor did we put limitations on caregivers, recognizing that they could include relatives, friends, or community members performing formal and informal, paid or unpaid work. Participants were asked to self-identify and were not required to provide proof of Indigenous ancestry. Using Indigenous research methodologies, we interviewed eighty Indigenous women, and although only eight discussed age-related dementia, their experiences of providing care were varied, and several common themes did arise during the study. The in-depth interviews and research circles informed our team of the challenges that caregivers face and their recommendations for improving the situation. Ensuring that their stories are heard lies at the very heart of this project.

Situating the Research

The Indigenous population of Canada is the fastest growing segment in the country, making up 4.3 percent of the total population (Statistics Canada 2011a). Although the median age of the Indigenous population as a whole is thirteen years younger than that of the general Canadian population, the number of Indigenous seniors doubled between 1996 and 2006 (Statistics Canada 2008). This increase may seem significant, but in 2011 Indigenous seniors aged sixty-five and over accounted for 5.9 percent of the total Indigenous population, whereas non-Indigenous seniors accounted for 14.2 percent of the population (Statistics Canada 2011a). Even though the health and well-being of Indigenous people has increased over the last fifty years, they still experience higher rates of ill health than non-Indigenous people.

Their health status is far below the national average. They die at a younger age and are plagued by higher rates of chronic diseases, cancers, and mental illnesses (Reading and Halseth 2013). It is important to note that, due to health disparities between Indigenous and non-Indigenous people in Canada, Indigenous people are considered seniors at the age of fifty-five years, as opposed to sixty-five for the general population (Canada 2009; Health Canada 1998; Health Council of Canada 2013). Available health surveillance data suggest that Indigenous people experience much higher rates of co-morbidities than their non-Indigenous counterparts. For example, the number of First Nations people aged fifty-five to sixty-four who report three or more chronic conditions is 3.5 times higher than for non–First Nations people. Forty-five percent of those who are sixty-five and older report fair/poor health, with 69 percent having activity limitations (Wilson, Rosenberg, and Abonyi 2011). It is generally accepted that poorer levels of health in the Indigenous population are deeply rooted in inequity, social exclusion, historical injustice, and the social determinants of health (Loppie Reading and Wein 2009).

There are many factors that put Indigenous people at risk for ill health, some of which include poverty, substandard housing, lack of access to health care, food insecurity, low levels of education, violence, and incarceration. Environmental factors, such as poor air and water quality, contribute as well. Living in poverty can diminish a person's ability to access nutritious foods, quality housing, and/or health care. This in turn can harm the physical and cognitive development of children and youth, and can impair the cognitive abilities of adults (National Collaborating Centre for Aboriginal Health 2010).

Aging is the most significant non-modifiable risk factor for the development of dementia (Alzheimer Society of Canada 2010). Population projections for Indigenous people suggest that though this group is still relatively young, the numbers of those who are fifty-five and older are growing. Given that aging is associated with dementia, we may expect that its prevalence among Indigenous seniors would be higher than among non-Indigenous seniors due to higher rates of chronic disease and greater exposure to risk factors (see Chapter 1, this volume). Further, dementia is often related to the presence of one or more chronic illnesses, such as diabetes, heart disease, and stroke, which are known to occur at higher frequencies in Indigenous populations (Health Council of Canada 2013; Public Health Agency of Canada 2018; Tjepkema et al. 2012).

Some studies suggest that dementia is probably under-diagnosed in Indigenous populations. As reviewed by Jennifer Walker and Kristen Jacklin in Chapter 1 of this volume, studies show that Indigenous people may wait for an average of five years before seeking a diagnosis for dementia, compared to two years for Euro-Americans (Dilworth-Anderson 2010). This delay may be related to a mistrust of the medical profession (Griffin-Pierce et al. 2008), inadequate access to health resources (Morgan et al. 2009; Weiner, Rossetti, and Harrah 2011), and culturally grounded beliefs that dementia is a natural part of life (Griffin-Pierce et al. 2008; Jacklin, Pace, and Warry 2015). Much of the recent research concerning understandings of dementia in Indigenous populations suggests that it is often viewed as natural (Hulko et al. 2010; Jacklin and Warry 2011, 2012; Lanting et al. 2011). There is also some indication among the Secwepemc communities in British Columbia that understandings of dementia have changed over time and that distinctions are increasingly made between dementia as a disease and dementia as natural (Hulko et al. 2010).

The presence of multiple morbidities and risk factors complicates the diagnosis and treatment of dementia, as well as caregiving requirements (Jacklin, Walker, and Shawande, 2013; Jacklin and Warry 2011). Often, the result is a lack of diagnosis, or late diagnosis, because the co-morbid condition is prioritized, which can limit treatment options and compound the complexity of patient care (Jacklin and Warry 2012). Research also suggests that diagnosis and treatment of dementia may be relatively recent (J.N. Henderson and L.C. Henderson 2002; Jacklin, Pace, and Warry 2015; Jacklin, Walker, and Shawande 2013), but they are also an increasing phenomenon (Chapter 1, this volume). In Canada, dementia rates for First Nations are reported to be 34 percent higher than for non–First Nations people; the same study revealed that First Nations individuals developed dementia at an earlier age and that it was most prevalent in males (Jacklin, Walker, and Shawande 2013).[3] Furthermore, rates are predicted to rise due to an increase in life expectancy "and the prevalence of risk factors for dementia such as diabetes, low socio-economic status and/or poverty, obesity, cardiovascular disease, and low levels of formal education" (Hulko et al. 2010, 318). This trend is set against the Canadian context, where the number of people with dementia or Alzheimer's disease is anticipated to expand from 480,618 in 2008 to 1,125,184 in 2038 (Alzheimer Society of Canada 2010). In Canada, the total economic burden of dementia and Alzheimer's, which includes direct health costs, opportunity costs of informal caregivers (lost wages), and indirect costs, was approximately $15 billion in 2008 and is expected to rise to $153 billion by 2038 (Alzheimer Society of Canada 2010). At present, Canada has no national strategy for dementia, though some provinces, such as Ontario and Quebec, have comprehensive plans in place to address the increasing numbers of dementia and Alzheimer's patients (Rockwood and Keren 2010).

Given these facts, we can anticipate that the aging Indigenous population will present serious challenges for health care systems, Indigenous communities, and caregivers. The burden of caring for a loved one who has dementia often falls on the family, as outside care and long-term-care facilities that will accept such a patient can be expensive and isolating, especially if the person is removed from his or her community (Kane and Houston-Vega 2004). In rural or remote areas, family care may be the only option that permits the person to remain in the community, as many First

Nations reserves have neither trained homecare staff nor suitable long-term-care facilities. This growing Indigenous senior population will present challenges to the health care system and caregivers, which will simply be exacerbated if professionals, families, and communities are not provided with timely and culturally appropriate information on dementia and its related diseases.

To enhance our understanding of the impacts of dementia on Indigenous individuals, families, and communities, we analyzed interview and research circle data that spoke to people's experiences with dementia and Alzheimer's. We were able to examine how the participants thought about and understood dementia, the impacts of caring for a loved one who had it, whether they felt there were gaps in support, and ultimately what they felt was needed to promote and support people with dementia, their families, and communities. Interviewers from the Understanding from Within (UFW) project spoke with six caregivers, many of whom were looking after a family member with dementia, and two health care providers, who shared insights on caring for people with dementia in the Canadian health care system. The unique insights and recommendations in these interviews provide a glimpse into the realities faced by caregivers, who often experience alienation, isolation, and a general lack of support from their community and the health care system.

A Select Review of the Literature

Though it was not comprehensive, our literature review found very few studies on Indigenous experiences with dementia and dementia care in Canada. Much of the research focuses on Native American populations of the southwest United States (Jervis, Boland, and Fickenscher 2010). Whereas several studies examine perceptions of dementia within Indigenous communities, formal care structures, and barriers to care, they only begin to address the vast gap in current knowledge. We found just one study that fully examined the role or experiences of informal caregivers for Indigenous populations in Canada. Other studies made only cursory references to Indigenous people in Canada. This lack is notable, given the comparably large dementia literature for other cultural or ethnic groups (such as the Chinese) and the frequent references to the important role that culture plays in determining experiences of caregiving and illness (Llanque and Enriquez 2012).

Several studies note the limitations of the current approach to dementia in the Indigenous population, which consists largely of interventions that are grounded in the experiences and conceptions of the "mainstream," mostly white, middle-class population (Hulko 2009). As Shawnda Lanting et al. (2011) observe, dementia care interventions for Indigenous people are difficult to design and provide without adequate knowledge of their community. One significant barrier to high-quality and successful care, from testing to long-term management, is the lack of culturally appropriate tools and conceptions of the illness (Lanting 2011; Lanting et al. 2011).

The standard approach to dementia, which is largely negative, concentrates on treating it as an illness. Several studies suggest, however, that this conception does not accurately reflect the heterogeneous nature of illness experience (Hulko 2009). Many studies discussed differing perceptions of dementia. The studies that examined participant ideas about dementia reported that they held varied and sometimes contradictory views. Some Indigenous individuals and communities saw dementia symptoms as a natural part of aging or an expected return to childhood (Cammer 2006; Finkelstein, Forbes, and Richmond 2012; Jacklin, Pace, and Warry 2015; Lanting et al. 2011). Another common theme was that dementia sprang from a change in culture and the degradation of traditional lifeways (Lanting et al. 2011). Several studies also observed that the communities they examined were generally unaware of dementia or knew little about it (Cammer 2006; Finkelstein, Forbes, and Richmond 2012; Lanting et al. 2011). Finally, whereas some Indigenous people saw dementia as normal or even spiritual, others perceived it as a source of embarrassment, fear, and shame (Cammer 2006; Finkelstein, Forbes, and Richmond 2012).

General factors affecting quality of care commonly include barriers associated with the isolation or low socioeconomic status of communities, such as transportation challenges, lack of resources and respite care, and a focus on crisis mitigation rather than long-term management (Finkelstein, Forbes, and Richmond 2012; Jacklin, Pace, and Warry 2015). The literature also cites additional factors as affecting both the identification of symptoms and experiences of illness and caregiving, including ways in which aging is viewed, differences in language, and general situational differences (Finkelstein, Forbes, and Richmond 2012; Lanting et al. 2011). Language, in particular, was mentioned: not only did it make communications with health care providers challenging, but it also affected the ways in which dementia was understood (Cammer 2006; Finkelstein, Forbes, and Richmond 2012). Additionally, differing perceptions of dementia complicate its diagnosis and treatment (Finkelstein, Forbes, and Richmond 2012; Lanting et al. 2011). As was widely observed, people who see dementia symptoms as natural are unlikely to seek care until a crisis occurs (Finkelstein, Forbes, and Richmond 2012). Similarly, stigma and embarrassment are strong barriers that prevent diagnosis and care (Cammer 2006; Finkelstein, Forbes, and Richmond 2012). Notably, as several studies pointed out, dementia was frequently not a priority in communities that were preoccupied with a multitude of other challenges, particularly when it did not directly interfere with daily functioning (Cammer 2006; Hulko 2009).

Furthermore, the lack of Indigenous-specific resources and acceptance was frequently identified in the literature as a significant, under-addressed, and multifaceted obstacle to care. The absence of First Nations–specific literature and outreach literature limited both formal and informal caregivers (Finkelstein, Forbes, and Richmond 2012; Jacklin, Pace, and Warry 2015). The lack of Indigenous-specific diagnostic tools is also noted as a barrier to care (Lanting et al. 2011). Finkelstein, Forbes, and Richmond (2012) found that a lack of First Nations–specific information on dementia inhibited careworkers' ability to communicate effectively with clients regarding memory function, especially the importance of early diagnosis. They stress the importance of the need for health care professionals to learn about the local cultural context and develop relationships with families and clients to ensure their approaches are appropriate (Finkelstein, Forbes, and Richmond 2012). Several studies also stress the importance of supporting traditional community caregiving and family caring for people with dementia, at home, for as long as possible (Jacklin, Pace, and Warry 2015; Lanting et al. 2011). A low rate of service access may also be potentially attributable to a deeply and historically embedded mistrust of health care and government (Jacklin et al. 2017).

Given the research to date, suggesting that dementia, including both the illness experience and broader community approaches, is highly influenced by specific culture and socioeconomic status, the need for further studies is evident. In particular, more research is needed regarding the dementia experiences of Canadian Indigenous people, especially those of specific stakeholders within communities, including informal caregivers (Finkelstein, Forbes, and Richmond 2012).

Conducting the Research

The NPHSNC consulted with experts from the Canadian neurological research community regarding which neurological conditions should be included in the study. It then selected fourteen conditions, basing its choice on the lack of knowledge concerning them and their potential burden on the population.[4] The UFW research team and advisory committee recognized that by limiting participation to Indigenous people who had one of the fourteen conditions or who cared for them, they would be silencing people who wanted their stories to be heard. Thus, we expanded our scope to encompass any condition that affected the brain, the spine, or the nervous system. As a result, we were able to speak with participants who had a condition that fell outside the original list or who cared for them. Relevant conditions here were Rett syndrome, ataxia, trigeminal neuralgia, Kennedy's disease, migraine, and stroke.

The UFW research team used a qualitative methodology, integrating Indigenous research methodologies (IRM) into the design of the questions, collection of data, and analysis of findings. This was done through incorporating the four Rs of research involving Indigenous people: respect, reciprocity, relevance, and responsibility (Kirkness and Barnhardt 1991). For some participants, this was the first opportunity to share their experiences. Given that research in many Indigenous communities has been neither relevant, reciprocal, nor conducted respectfully, we felt it imperative that the stories told to us should be shared in a meaningful way.

To ensure that the research was respectful and relevant to the experiences of Indigenous people throughout Canada, the UFW research team established an advisory committee, which consisted of two Elders, two youth, and six Indigenous and non-Indigenous specialists from across the country who had worked closely within Indigenous health and research.[5] The committee helped guide the research, assisted with the recruitment process, and performed data analysis. The UFW research team took a four-directional approach in recruiting participants, working closely with advisory committee members from each of these areas so that IRM protocols were followed. The advisory committee members advised the UFW research team of the area-specific protocols that needed to be followed to ensure that the process was culturally sensitive, safe, and relevant for all participants. The advisory committee members also provided guidance to the research team and served as liaisons in contacting communities, setting up research circles, and addressing participants' questions or concerns. The advisory committee as a whole provided valuable feedback on research design, data collection, and analysis, and grounded the research in traditional cultural teachings and Western academic standards. These steps ensured that the research was conducted in a culturally appropriate and responsible manner.

To enable participants to share their stories fully, the UFW research team used two methods: in-depth interviews and research circles (focus groups). Participants could choose the method they preferred, whether it was a one-on-one interview or the group setting of a circle. During the interviews and circles, they were offered food, refreshments, and a small honorarium for sharing their knowledge and experiences. Transportation and childcare were also provided for those who otherwise could not have participated. The UFW interviewers explained the details of the project, including how they themselves became involved, where they were from, and their own experiences with neurological conditions. This process of sharing personal information is consistent with IRM in terms of building relationships.

In-depth interviews were conducted with three groups: eighteen key informants (KI), made up of Indigenous and non-Indigenous health care professionals; four traditional knowledge holders (TKH), consisting of Elders and healers; and seventeen individuals (ID) – Indigenous people who had a neurological condition or who cared for someone who did. Participants, also referred to as "co-researchers" in the spirit of reciprocity and collaborative research, were asked three open-ended questions, which differed slightly from group to group. Interviews could last anywhere from 45 to 150 minutes.

Research circles were also used to share and gather knowledge. We held six research circles in three provinces and one territory, with a total of forty-one participants. Following IRM, the UFW team worked closely with a community contact person to ensure that the circles were culturally appropriate. Where suitable, the team presented Elders with tobacco, cloth, and an honorarium, and asked them to open and close the circle with a prayer. In so doing, the team was asking for prayers that the research would be conducted in a good way; for the health and well-being of the participants and the strength and courage that they embodied in sharing their stories; and for the team itself to not only hear these incredible stories, but to work with them in a way that showed respect and that honoured the manner in which they were told. Adhering to community protocols is necessary if research circles are to be relevant to the people involved and to be conducted in a responsible manner.

Just as in a sharing circle, each participant told his or her story and then surrendered the floor to the next person. Depending on the number of participants, circles typically lasted for two to three hours, though two took more than four hours to complete.

Participants in both the interviews and the circles were asked the following questions:

- Prior to your experience with a neurological condition, what did you know or think about neurological health? How has your understanding of neurological health changed since diagnosis?
- What kind of impacts has the condition had on you or your family – for example, emotionally, spiritually, mentally, physically?
- In trying to develop a vision that comes from Indigenous women themselves to help guide ongoing and future efforts to foster neurological and overall health and well-being of Indigenous women, their families, and communities, we would like to ask you what you feel is needed, what you think would help to promote and support neurological health and well-being for Indigenous people and communities across Canada.

These questions were designed to allow participants to share their stories. Some had never fully told them before. We wanted to honour their voices, strengths, and experiences.

The interviews and research circles were recorded and transcribed, with a copy of the transcription being sent to participants for review. In this, they could choose from various options: a hard copy with a prepaid envelope could be mailed to their address, and they could mark it up and send it back; they could receive an electronic copy, which they could edit via track changes or comments and then email back; or an exact audio copy of the interview burned onto a compact disc could be mailed to them, along with a toll-free number that they could call to discuss any changes. The third option was available only to interviewees because audio extraction for the circles was not feasible at that time. Everyone was given the toll-free number and encouraged to call the UFW research team to go through the transcripts and discuss changes by October 2012 (prior to data analysis). After this date, all identifying information was removed from the transcripts, and the data were coded using NVivo 10. The UFW research team undertook the first phase of analysis, during which the initial themes and subthemes were isolated.

To uphold IRM, the advisory committee was invited to take part in the second phase of collective analysis, using an adapted collective consensual data analytic procedure, as described by Judith Bartlett et al. (2007). This process ensured that the findings remained relevant and that the advisory committee was included in a respectful way.[6] Major themes and subthemes emerged in the research, along with recommendations that were intended to improve relations between the medical community and Indigenous people, and to promote the importance of Indigenous control of health care services (NWAC 2013). A breakdown of the themes and subthemes can be found in the Appendix.

This chapter draws on individual interviews with two caregivers, key informant interviews with two health care professionals, and research circle stories shared by four caregivers. One individual interviewee looked after his mother, who had Alzheimer's disease, diabetes, and arthritis, whereas the other looked after her brother, who had HIV-related dementia and hepatitis C. None of the interviewees had Alzheimer's or any other form of dementia. All four circle participants provided care for someone who had dementia. The analysis that follows is based on interviews with six caregivers (First Nations and Métis) and two non-Indigenous health care providers.

Learning from the Participants Stories

Of the eighty participants in the UFW project, only eight discussed age-related dementia. The experiences of providing care were varied, but several common themes did arise during the study. The in-depth interviews and research circles informed us of the challenges that caregivers faced and their recommendations for improving the situation. Ensuring that their stories are heard lies at the very heart of this project.

Lack of Knowledge of Dementia and Stigmatization

An overarching theme was that caregivers and their communities were often poorly informed regarding dementia. Some participants linked this lack of information to delay in seeking medical care and diagnosis. For many participants, dementia was not identified as being at the forefront of their medical concerns. As one caregiver shared,

> So, as her symptoms increased, you know, I think it was denial, like, as the way that we kind of just put it off to that this is [what happens when you] age. You know, something that would be normally coming with aging. So, one of the things that she, and my younger sister noticed that because my mother had plants in her house and slowly, she kind of became, she didn't clean up as often in her house. She

didn't water her plants. So it became very obvious then that they needed to do something. And there were times when she would burn food. And that was really not, she wasn't a cook, but these were kind of just little things beginning to show, reveal themselves to us. (ID0726)

Many caregivers said that they were unfamiliar with the signs or symptoms of Alzheimer's and dementia. When these appeared, they simply concluded that their loved one was getting older and needing more assistance. Only when the symptoms became problematic did they start to ask for help or begin researching the condition.

Caregivers shouldered the daunting task of looking after increasingly ill friends or relatives who had developed an illness that they and the people around them knew little about. Notably, this was mentioned by individuals who were caring for relatives and by the professional care providers. Participants cited the lack of readily available information and the necessity of undertaking research independently.

An inability on the part of family and community members to understand the nature of dementia can isolate both patient and caregiver. One caregiver recalled that when his mother's symptoms started to progress, many of her relatives stopped coming to visit because they did not want to see her deteriorate:

I don't think they understood, and my younger sister was in denial, whereas once I think she understood what was going on with Mother ... She was the youngest sibling and she had two children or three, and once she realized what her, my mother had, she just had nothing to do with her. Like, she literally could not do it. So, she just stopped seeing my mother and just [had] no contact with Mother as a way of dealing with it, really not in a way dealing, but I doubt, and I think it was too much for her, like, emotionally or mentally, that it was [too hard] to see my mother like that, she just couldn't. (ID0726)

This greatly affected his relationship with his sister in that he could not rely on her to provide support of any kind, leaving him feeling alone and overburdened.

Individuals who experience memory loss are increasingly isolated not only by their condition, but also by the family or the community's failure to understand its nature. Further, due to these misunderstandings and the commitment required of the caregivers, the caregivers also felt a sense of being alone.

Several caregivers also mentioned the stigmatization and increased vulnerability of the individuals for whom they cared. One, whose brother was living with HIV-related dementia, described his difficulties with law enforcement and with people in general:

> So, I called the police and let them know that my brother has dementia and that he's not well, but I will come to get him the next day. I didn't want the police to pick him [up] and throw him in jail because he's been to jail, [and] that's not where he belongs, [as] he has a condition. People are afraid of him, but it's my brother that needs to be protected from others that want to hurt him. (IDo517)

Stigmatization can sometimes be difficult to disentangle from discrimination. The same participant made this point in connection with her efforts to arrange care for her brother: "My brother was on a waiting list for the homecare facilities here, but I believe that they don't want him there because he's a First Nation and HIV-positive and probably not because of the dementia" (IDo517).

Personal Difficulties Faced by Caregivers

Another theme that emerged in the interviews and circles was the personal difficulties of the caregivers. In addition to being Indigenous, many struggled with their health, substance abuse in their families, financial problems, lack of stable support structures, and multiple caregiving responsibilities. As many observed, dementia was just one of the numerous challenges in their lives. Although they willingly accepted their role and recognized its importance to the well-being of the person whom they looked after, it came with a multitude of challenges. One participant mentioned the difficulty of caring for someone who had a variety of co-morbidities: "And I noticed he'd have his medication because he's on medication – he's diabetic – he'd have his pills in the garbage; he'd throw them away. I said, 'How come those are in the garbage?' [And he said] 'I don't need them; I don't need them'" (research circle 0821).

Several participants spoke of missing work or being unemployed because caregiving consumed so much of their time. Looking after someone who might need round-the-clock attention made it difficult and physically tiring to hold down a job as well. Several individuals said they felt emotionally and spiritually drained by the demands of caregiving, especially considering the lack of support that many mentioned.

In addition to feeling sad or frustrated by watching dementia diminish their loved one, several participants also felt guilty because they could not fully care for the person. One woman who looked after her mother said, "I think emotionally it's just tearing me apart [and] spiritually [it's] probably just as bad. And [there's] just a lot of guilt and you can't carry it all for her you know, it's hard" (research circle 0522).

Understandings and Interpretations of a Neurological Condition

However, not all the comments were negative. One participant, a registered nurse, spoke about differing interpretations of dementia: "Yes, one person's spiritual enlightenment is another person's pathology. It's true in every culture, not just in First Nations culture. It's also a matter of context – look at Joan of Arc or people who claim to speak to God" (KI0516).

No one else discussed cultural conceptions of dementia and neurological conditions, but several people commented on memory loss and dementia symptoms as a normal part of aging. Many cared for order adults and saw memory loss as an aspect of becoming old, albeit a difficult one: "It just seems that we accept an illness as part of life and deal with it individually or [as] a part of the equation" (ID0726).

Nonetheless, participants wished that they had a better understanding of care and preventative measures, especially those who had looked after someone with late-stage diagnosed dementia. Several observed that, due to pride and a desire for privacy, their older family members often did not discuss new symptoms when they arose. Notably, a registered nurse also said, "People who are hungry and do not have a place to sleep are going to be consumed by those basic needs before they can even address their neurological health. People will naturally think about only those primary needs and only when those are met will they come forward" (KI0516).

This viewpoint was indirectly supported by the stories of many participants, who, when asked about experiences with neurological conditions, listed the vast array of medical issues faced by their family, several of which were far more immediate than neurology. The symptoms that cause the most pain will be addressed first, and neurological conditions that may exhibit no painful symptoms will become a lower priority.

Experiences with the Health Care System

In discussing the health care system and the available supports, participants identified several areas of concern and recommended improvements. Many emphasized easy access to information and educational opportunities as a crucial part of improving dementia care and noted that the system was falling short in this respect. Several found that doctors could be uninformative, providing only the most basic information. One stated, "No medical professional has explained the progression of the condition. I have had to do research on my own about his condition online in any free time that I have, but I don't have much opportunity to do so" (ID0517).

Interactions with doctors and health care providers were limited and, for some, infrequent. Several participants saw hospitals and medical attention as a last resort, taken only when it became unavoidable. As a result, care was often sought late in the illness, and diagnoses were delayed until an event requiring hospitalization occurred. Several participants mentioned the need for further public education and awareness, to encourage individuals to seek medical care when symptoms appeared and to reduce stigma throughout the community.

Participants also suggested that people were reluctant to access the health system because it lacked a traditional Indigenous medicine option. Accompanying this dissatisfaction was a sense that current health structures failed to take a holistic approach to the needs of individuals with dementia and their caregivers. The care provided addressed only the physical aspect of well-being and tended to neglect the emotional and spiritual aspects: "They kind of compartmentalize health, you know, we still say holistic health from our visits. You get these experts, but it's almost like it's a neurological disease. Even though the brain is so imperative to who we are, it's still not seen as a priority" (ID0726).

Participants strongly recommended the inclusion of services that treated dementia holistically and considered the person as a whole. Several suggested that traditional treatment options and foods be offered in care homes. A registered nurse stated that health professionals should be educated regarding the value of traditional approaches and the need for further research.

Finally, participants overwhelmingly recommended that support systems and counselling be put in place for caregivers, friends, and families. Many mentioned the difficulty of meeting with others in comparable situations.

Similarly, several expressed a desire for more readily available and affordable formal counselling. As one stated,

> I guess what I would like to see at a community level would be more support groups or a sharing circle [so] that families who experience it can get together. Because you know not everyone is alone and everyone, like, most families suffer from some sort of neurological disorder I guess. (research circle 0522)

Support groups were seen as a means of education, of addressing unmet emotional needs, and of generating solidarity. Several participants said that the development of such groups would minimize the isolation of caregivers. Of all the recommendations they made, the need to provide mutual support within communities was voiced most strongly.

Understanding the Importance of Dementia Research with Indigenous People

Co-morbidities, Complexity of Care, and the Low Prioritization of Dementia

As mentioned above, only eight of the eighty participants in the UFW study spoke about dementia. This in itself was a surprising finding that led to some speculation among the research team. Under-diagnosis, differing views on the nature of aging, and the low prioritization of dementia may all contribute to a lack of awareness or discussion of the subject within Indigenous communities. These factors, coupled with possible stigma or discrimination, may explain the relative silence regarding dementia.

For those who did discuss it, dementia occurred within a complex set of circumstances; for example, caregivers reported the concurrence of diabetes, arthritis, HIV, and hepatitis C. Dementia complicates the management of co-morbidities, as memory loss, the inability to perform tasks, and the difficulty of comprehending ideas make taking medications, seeking medical assistance, and navigating the health care system exponentially more difficult (Maslow 2004). In addition, given the high presence and pressing nature of co-morbidities in Indigenous populations, as in the case of diabetes, it is likely that dementia is not prioritized (Jacklin and Warry 2012). Thus, for caregivers and individuals, it becomes "the last issue on the list." It is often undiagnosed, partly because other conditions take precedence and partly because, as reviewed, some Indigenous people may not recognize it as a disease or identify the symptoms and therefore would not seek care (Finkelstein, Forbes, and Richmond 2012; Jacklin, Pace, and Warry 2015; Lanting et al. 2011). Since dementia can complicate the management of other conditions, its early diagnosis is essential, so that care, treatment, and measures to slow its progress can be discussed. Yet, studies have noted the many barriers at play here, such as geography, health policy, and mistrust of health care systems (Finkelstein, Forbes, and Richmond 2012; Jacklin, Pace, and Warry 2015). To offset these, it is important to devise culturally safe methods of building awareness among caregivers and in communities to ensure that Indigenous people know how to access dementia-related information and services and feel comfortable when doing so. This can help them make decisions about dementia treatment and care that are informed by their own cultural values and what Western medicine may offer.

Supportive Services and Respite Care

Supportive services and respite care were a common theme for care providers throughout the larger NWAC project, and they were a key theme among the participants who discussed dementia (NWAC 2013). These individuals revealed that acquiring homecare is a problem for many people in rural, northern, or remote areas. In these locales, accessing culturally appropriate respite services and day programs can be difficult for Indigenous seniors generally and for those with dementia. This lack of respite is a common finding (Finkelstein, Forbes, and Richmond 2012). The participants who were discussed in Jacklin, Pace, and Warry (2015) mentioned the need for respite that would be "appropriate" for Indigenous families.

In capturing the experiences of looking after a loved one with dementia, the UFW project offers insights into how caregivers are affected by poor or restricted access to services. These individuals tend to be the ones who discuss care plans with physicians and other health care providers, and they are key advocates. Among our participants, they were typically family members who reported multiple hardships. They were not paid for their services, and they often faced financial challenges, missed work, or were unemployed because caregiving took up so much of their time. Looking after someone with dementia was taxing, and as a result they felt physically, emotionally, mentally, and spiritually drained. Many cited the lack of support and felt guilty because they could not fully satisfy their numerous responsibilities. Other studies document the challenges of caring for a person with dementia and also elucidate Indigenous-specific coping strategies and the benefits of family caregiving (Botsford, Clarke, and Gibb 2011; Jacklin, Pace, and Warry 2015; Jervis, Boland, and Fickenscher 2010).

Addressing Dementia Knowledge and Experience

Information and knowledge needs surrounding dementia emerged as a cross-cutting theme. Family caregivers referred to their own lack of knowledge and experience with dementia as a factor that limited their ability to care for a person who had the condition. They also said that physicians and health care workers provided little to no information on the illness, obliging them to research it on their own. There was also a notable lack of experiential knowledge concerning dementia. Significantly, one family caregiver described it as "a whole new realm," which may support the notion that it is an emerging illness in Indigenous populations (Cammer 2006; J.N. Henderson and L.C. Henderson 2002; Jacklin and Warry 2012). Clearly, for these participants, not understanding the biomedical dimensions of the disease was related to not knowing how to provide care or how to access appropriate services. Research with non-Indigenous populations shows that family caregivers who do not receive adequate training and support regarding dementia are at a high risk for adverse effects, such as burnout, and will provide low quality care (Kokkonen et al. 2013; Williamson, Shaffer, and Family Relationship in Late Life Project 2001). Family caregiving is extremely common in Indigenous communities (Buchignani and Armstrong-Esther 1999; Korn et al. 2009), suggesting that the education and training of family caregivers is essential.

Related to this, our work and that of others (Hulko 2009; Hulko et al. 2010; Jacklin, Pace, and Warry 2015; Lanting et al. 2011) suggest that elements of cultural safety also permeate the dementia experience for caregivers. The stories of UFW participants suggest that some aspects of the dementia experience are unique to Indigenous people, including cultural understandings of the illness as natural or spiritual, holistic versus compartmentalized views of the brain, and negative interaction with the health care system that is related to colonization. Although the eight people who discussed dementia did not speak to issues of historical trauma and historical experiences with the health care system, this theme did emerge in the larger dataset (see Appendix) and has been found in other studies (Jacklin, Pace, and Warry 2015). These findings, along with the work of others, suggest that educational information and programs for Indigenous people must be grounded in contextual knowledge.

Implications

Although only a few UFW participants discussed Alzheimer's disease or dementia, some important issues did emerge. Our findings add to the growing body of literature on dementia in Indigenous communities that shows the need for a greater emphasis on this condition in the health care setting. Specifically, participants recommended that awareness regarding dementia be improved in their communities to minimize misconceptions and maximize care. They suggested that support systems and counselling be implemented for caregivers and families, and for individuals experiencing dementia. They also called for the creation of support groups to diminish the isolation that many caregivers felt.

The larger-scale distribution of information to Indigenous communities would also seem essential, as participants mentioned that the inability of family and community members to understand dementia led to the isolation of both patient and caregiver. They recommended that more accessible information be made available in communities and that health care providers take a more holistic approach to care. Importantly, education and information should be provided in a way that is culturally safe and meaningful to the community. This necessitates the inclusion of traditional Indigenous health approaches and cultural understandings of dementia. Having an Indigenous advisory committee to assist with the development of educational resources could help expand the dialogue between health care providers and Indigenous people. Training health care workers in cultural safety may encourage Indigenous people to interact more regularly with care services. Providing culturally relevant services in a safe, compassionate manner could improve both care-seeking behaviour and the experience of health care for the patient. Cultural safety training is currently offered at the university level in nursing, public health, and medicine programs (Baba 2013). In communities where the number of dementia patients is growing, it could aid them to generate their own solutions, based on best practices from other communities. Participants also recommended further public education, awareness, and training to reduce stigma. The participants also noted that awareness campaigns are useful only when supportive services are in place and are adequate to meet community needs. Finally, the lack of awareness and under-diagnosis points to the need for more targeted, community-based research with Indigenous people and for their inclusion in any talks concerning a national dementia strategy.

The UFW study, along with others in this volume and elsewhere, provides some valuable information regarding dementia among Indigenous people, but clearly much more research must be done with, by, and for them. The truth is that they are the ones who experience these issues on a daily basis and are therefore best equipped to guide this research. Health care providers certainly have a role to play in confronting stigma and discrimination and in creating culturally safe service delivery, but the Indigenous communities themselves must lead the research, which must be relevant, useful, and action-oriented. We hope that this information will help spark the conversations that will bring about the necessary change and provide support for Indigenous caregivers, families, and individuals experiencing dementia and other neurological diseases.

Released in 2015, the report of the Truth and Reconciliation Commission of Canada (TRC 2015) includes recommendations that are intended to improve the health care system and close the gap in health outcomes for Indigenous people. Tellingly, the suggestions of many UFW participants align with those of the commission:

i.   Increase the number of Aboriginal professionals working in the health-care field.
ii. Ensure the retention of Aboriginal health-care providers in Aboriginal communities.
iii. Provide cultural competency training for all health-care professionals. (TRC 2015, 3)

Given that dementia is on the rise among Indigenous communities, they must play a role in the creation of any national strategy to address it, especially but by no means limited to cultural understandings of the disease.

❖ ❖ ❖

Our findings, along with a growing body of literature on dementia in Indigenous people, are peppered with deep experiences of health inequity, systemic barriers to health care, and the need for better supports.

The analysis of the UFW stories enables us to situate a portion of our data in the emerging field of Indigenous dementia research. As is the case for many diseases, examining the dementia experience of Indigenous people illuminates the health inequity that typifies their lives, including ongoing marginalization and systemic barriers to care. On a purely practical level, we argue that the findings point to the need for better access to information, better supports for caregivers, and better management of patients with co-morbidities.

Appendix: UFW Summary of Analytic Categories

Major themes	Subthemes
Challenges and recommendations	Fighting for rights; Non-Insured Health Benefits (NIHB); recommendations for health care providers; recommendations for policy
Circle of support	Caregiver experiences; community issues; impact of friends; lack of support; support; support groups
Colonial and systemic factors	Abuse; discrimination; environmental factors; intergenerational impacts; stigma; trauma
Disease process (pathology)	Conditions; diagnosis; medication; symptoms; treatment
Impacts of neurological conditions	Community impacts; educational impacts; family impacts; financial impacts; housing impacts; mental impacts; mobility impacts; physical impacts; social determinants of health; spiritual impacts; work and career impacts
Interaction with the health care system	Access to health care; culturally relevant care; health care gaps; homecare; ability to navigate; negligence of care; positive health care experience; respite
Knowledge and information	Communication issues; information needs about neurological conditions; knowledge gaps; knowledge of health care providers
Risks and protective factors	Co-morbidities; conditions; healthy self-care; injury; lifestyle; predisposition; resiliency
Traditions and culture	Alternative medicine; cultural influences; self-reflection; traditional approaches to healing; traditional ways of knowing

Acknowledgments

We would like to thank the Native Women's Association of Canada, the communities, the focus groups, the participants, the key informants, the traditional knowledge holders, and the UFW advisory committee. We were humbled and honoured by the stories shared with us during the UFW project. Funding for the project was provided by the Public Health Agency of Canada as part of the National Population Health Study of Neurological Conditions.

Notes

1   The full title of the project was "Understanding from Within (UFW): Developing Community Driven and Culturally-Relevant Models for Understanding and Responding to Neurological Conditions among Aboriginal Peoples." The authors were involved in the larger Understanding from Within Project through the following roles: Carrie Bourassa was the principal investigator; Melissa Blind was the research co-ordinator; Kristen Jacklin was an advisory committee member; and Eric Oleson was a research assistant. Kate Ross-Hopley, who assisted with this chapter, was a research assistant during a practicum placement in the summer of 2014. Note that an advisory committee played a key role in the UFW research project and comprised Elders, knowledge keepers, and Indigenous and non-Indigenous experts in the field.

2   Note that when the project was under way, from 2011 to March 31, 2013, dementia was classified as a neurological condition. This definition was changed in May 2013, under the *Diagnostic and Statistical Manual of Mental Disorders* (DSM-5), to a neurocognitive disorder.

3   We use "First Nations" here instead of "Aboriginal" because the relevant data are registry data and are First Nations–specific.

4   The fourteen conditions were Alzheimer's disease and related dementia, amyotrophic lateral sclerosis, brain tumours, cerebral palsy, dystonia, epilepsy, Huntington disease, hydrocephalus, multiple sclerosis, muscular dystrophy, neurotrauma, Parkinson's disease, spina bifida, and Tourette syndrome.

5   For a complete listing of the UFW team and advisory committee members, please refer to NWAC (2013).

6   For more information on this process, see NWAC (2013).

References

Alzheimer Society of Canada. 2010. "Rising Tide: The Impact of Dementia on Canadian Society." http://alzheimer.ca/sites/default/files/files/chapters-on/york/rising_tide_full_report_eng_final.pdf.

Baba, Lauren. 2013. *Cultural Safety in First Nations, Inuit and Métis Public Health: Environmental Scan of Cultural Competency and Safety in Education, Training and Health Services.* Prince George, BC: National Collaborating Centre for Aboriginal Health. https://www.ccnsa-nccah.ca/docs/emerging/RPT-CulturalSafetyPublic Health-Baba-EN.pdf.

Bartlett, Judith G., Yoshitaka Iwasaki, Benjamin Gottlieb, Darlene Hall, and Roger Mannell. 2007. "Framework for Aboriginal-Guided Decolonizing Research Involving Métis and First Nations Persons with Diabetes." *Social Science and Medicine* 65 (11): 2371–82.

Botsford, Julia, Charlotte L. Clarke, and Catherine E. Gibb. 2011. "Research and Dementia, Caring and Ethnicity: A Review of the Literature." *Journal of Research in Nursing* 16 (5): 437–49.

Buchignani, Norman, and Christopher Armstrong-Esther. 1999. "Informal Care and Older Native Canadians." *Ageing and Society* 19 (1): 3–32.

Cammer, Allison Lee. 2006. "Negotiating Culturally Incongruent Healthcare Systems: The Process of Accessing Dementia Care in Northern Saskatchewan." Master's thesis, University of Saskatchewan. http://hdl.handle.net/10388/etd-12192006-160831.

Canada. Special Senate Committee on Aging. 2009. *Canada's Aging Population: Seizing the Opportunity*. Final report. https://sencanada.ca/content/sen/Committee/402/agei/rep/AgingFinalReport-e.pdf.

Dilworth-Anderson, Peggye. 2010. "Diagnosis of Alzheimer's within Cultural Context." *Alzheimer's and Dementia* 6 (4): S95.

Finkelstein, S.A., D.A. Forbes, and C.A. Richmond. 2012. "Formal Dementia Care among First Nations in Southwestern Ontario." *Canadian Journal on Aging* 31 (3): 257–70.

First Nations Regional Health Survey. N.d. "Fact Sheet: The Health and Wellbeing of Women in First Nations Communities." http://fnigc.ca/sites/default/files/ENpdf/RHS_2002/FN_Womens_Forum_Fact_Sheet.pdf.

Griffin-Pierce, Trudy, Nina Silverberg, Donald Connor, Minnie Jim, Jill Peters, Alfred Kaszniak, and Marwan N. Sabbagh. 2008. "Challenges to the Recognition and Assessment of Alzheimer's Disease in American Indians of the Southwestern United States." *Alzheimer's and Dementia: The Journal of the Alzheimer's Association* 4 (4): 291–99. DOI:10.1016/j.jalz.2007.10.012.

Health Canada. 1998. *Reaching Out: A Guide to Communicating with Aboriginal Seniors*. Ottawa: Division of Aging and Seniors, Health Canada. http://publications.gc.ca/collections/Collection/H88-3-20-1998E.pdf.

Health Council of Canada. 2013. "Canada's Most Vulnerable: Improving Health Care for First Nations, Inuit, and Métis Seniors." http://www.hhr-rhs.ca/images/stories/Senior_AB_Report_2013_EN_final.pdf.

Henderson, J. Neil, and L. Carson Henderson. 2002. "Cultural Construction of Disease: A 'Supernormal' Construct of Dementia in an American Indian Tribe." *Journal of Cross-Cultural Gerontology* 17 (3): 197–212.

Hennessy, Catherine Hagan, and Robert John. 1995. "The Interpretation of Burden among Pueblo Indian Caregivers." *Journal of Aging Studies* 9 (3): 215–29.

—. 1996. "American Indian Family Caregivers' Perceptions of Burden and Needed Support Services." *Journal of Applied Gerontology* 15 (3): 275–93. DOI:10.1177/073346489601500301.

Hulko, Wendy. 2009. "From 'Not a Big Deal' to 'Hellish': Experiences of Older People with Dementia." *Journal of Aging Studies* 23 (3): 131–44. DOI:10.1016/j.jaging.2007.11.002.

Hulko, Wendy, Evelyn Camille, Elisabeth Antifeau, Mike Arnouse, Nicole Bachynksi, and Denise Taylor. 2010. "Views of First Nation Elders on Memory Loss and Memory Care in Later Life." *Journal of Cross-Cultural Gerontology* 25 (4): 317–42.

Jacklin, Kristen M., Rita I. Henderson, Michael E. Green, Leah M. Walker, Betty

Calam, and Lynden J. Crowshoe. 2017. "Health Care Experiences of Indigenous People Living with Type 2 Diabetes in Canada." *Canadian Medical Association Journal* 189 (3): E106–12. DOI:10.1503/cmaj.161098.

Jacklin, Kristen, Jessica E. Pace, and Wayne Warry. 2015. "Informal Dementia Caregiving among Indigenous Communities in Ontario, Canada." *Care Management Journals* 16 (2): 106–20. DOI:10.1891/1521-0987.16.2.106.

Jacklin, Kristen M., Jennifer D. Walker, and Marjory Shawande. 2013. "The Emergence of Dementia as a Health Concern among First Nations Populations in Alberta, Canada." *Canadian Journal of Public Health* 104 (1): e39–e44. DOI:10.17269/cjph .104.3348.

Jacklin, Kristen, and Wayne Warry. 2011. "Diverse Experiences: Perspectives on Alzheimer's Disease in Aboriginal Communities in Ontario." Paper presented at the Alzheimer's Disease International Conference, Toronto, ON. http://www.alz .co.uk/adi-conference-2011-presentations.

–. 2012. "Forgetting and Forgotten: Dementia in Aboriginal Seniors." *Anthropology and Aging Quarterly* 33: 13.

Jervis, Lori L., Mathew E. Boland, and Alexandra Fickenscher. 2010. "American Indian Family Caregivers' Experiences with Helping Elders." *Journal of Cross-Cultural Gerontology* 25 (4): 355–69.

Kane, Michael N., and Mary Kay Houston-Vega. 2004. "Maximizing Content on Elders with Dementia while Teaching Multicultural Diversity." *Journal of Social Work Education* 40 (2): 285–303.

Kirkness, Verna J., and Ray Barnhardt. 1991. "First Nations and Higher Education: The Four R's – Respect, Relevance, Reciprocity, Responsibility." *Journal of American Indian Education* 30 (3): 1–15.

Kokkonen, Taru-Maija, Richard I.L. Cheston, Rudi Dallos, and Cordet A. Smart. 2013. "Attachment and Coping of Dementia Care Staff: The Role of Staff Attachment Style, Geriatric Nursing Self-Efficacy, and Approaches to Dementia in Burnout." *Dementia* 13 (4): 544–68.

Korn, Leslie, Rebecca G. Logsdon, Nayak L. Polissar, Alfredo Gomez-Beloz, Tiffany Waters, and Rudolph Rÿser. 2009. "A Randomized Trial of a CAM Therapy for Stress Reduction in American Indian and Alaskan Native Family Caregivers." *Gerontologist* 49 (3): 368–77.

Lanting, Shawnda. 2011. "Developing an Assessment Protocol to Detect Cognitive Impairment and Dementia in Cree Aboriginal Seniors and to Investigate Cultural Differences in Cognitive Aging." PhD diss., University of Saskatchewan. http://hdl .handle.net/10388/etd-04152011-143435.

Lanting, Shawnda, Margaret Crossley, Debra Morgan, and Alison Cammer. 2011. "Aboriginal Experiences of Aging and Dementia in a Context of Sociocultural Change: Qualitative Analysis of Key Informant Group Interviews with Aboriginal Seniors." *Journal of Cross-Cultural Gerontology* 26 (1): 103–17. DOI:10.1007/ s10823-010-9136-4.

Llanque, Sarah M., and Maithe Enriquez. 2012. "Interventions for Hispanic Caregivers of Patients with Dementia: A Review of the Literature." *American Journal of*

Alzheimer's Disease and Other Dementias 27 (1): 23–32.

Loppie Reading, Charlotte, and Fred Wein. 2009. *Health Inequalities and Social Determinants of Aboriginal Peoples' Health*. Prince George, BC: National Collaborating Centre for Aboriginal Health. http://www.nccah-ccnsa.ca/docs /social%20determinates/NCCAH-Loppie-Wien_Report.pdf.

Maslow, Katie. 2004. "Dementia and Serious Coexisting Medical Conditions: A Double Whammy." *Nursing Clinics of North America* 39 (3): 561–79. DOI:10.1016/j.cnur .2004.02.011.

Morgan, Debra G., et al. 2009. "Improving Access to Dementia Care: Development and Evaluation of a Rural and Remote Memory Clinic." *Aging and Mental Health* 13 (1): 17–30.

National Collaborating Centre for Aboriginal Health. 2010. "Poverty as a Social Determinant of First Nations, Inuit, and Métis Health." https://www.ccnsa-nccah. ca/docs/determinants/FS-PovertySDOH-EN.pdf.

NWAC (Native Women's Association of Canada). 2013. "Understanding from Within: Research Findings and NWAC's Contributions to Canada's National Population Health Study on Neurological Conditions (NPHSNC)."

Public Health Agency of Canada. 2018. "Social Determinants of Health and Health Inequalities" https://www.canada.ca/en/public-health/services/health-promotion /population-health/what-determines-health.html#wb-cont.

Reading, Jeff, and Regine Halseth. 2013. *Pathways to Improving Well-Being for Indigenous Peoples: How Living Conditions Decide Health*. Prince George, BC: National Collaborating Centre for Aboriginal Health. https://www.ccnsa-nccah.ca/docs/ determinants/RPT-PathwaysWellBeing-Reading-Halseth-EN.pdf.

Rockwood, Kenneth, and Ron Keren. 2010. "Dementia Services in Canada." *International Journal of Geriatric Psychiatry* 25 (9): 876–80. DOI:10.1002/gps.2590.

Statistics Canada. 2008. "2006 Census: Aboriginal Peoples in Canada in 2006: Inuit, Metis, and First Nations, 2006 Census." https://www12.statcan.gc.ca/census-recensement/2006/as-sa/97-558/p4-eng.cfm.

–. 2011a. "Aboriginal Peoples in Canada: First Nations People, Métis and Inuit." Catalogue No. 99-011-X2011001. https://www12.statcan.gc.ca/nhs-enm/2011/as-sa/99-011-x/99-011-x2011001-eng.cfm.

–. 2011b. "Canadian Community Health Survey." http://www.statcan.gc.ca/daily -quotidien/110621/dq110621b-eng.htm.

Tjepkema, M., R. Wilkins, N. Goedhuis, and J. Pennock. 2012. "Cardiovascular Disease Mortality among First Nations People in Canada, 1991–2001." *Chronic Diseases and Injuries in Canada* 32 (4): 200–7.

TRC (Truth and Reconciliation Commission of Canada). 2015. *The Truth and Reconciliation Commission of Canada: Calls to Action*. Winnipeg: TRC. http://nctr. ca/assets/reports/Calls_to_Action_English2.pdf.

Weiner, Myron F., Heidi C. Rossetti, and Kasia Harrah. 2011. "Videoconference Diagnosis and Management of Choctaw Indian Dementia Patients." *Alzheimer's and Dementia* 7 (6): 562–66.

Williamson, Gail M., David R. Shaffer, and The Family Relationships in Late Life Project. 2001. "Relationship Quality and Potentially Harmful Behaviours by Spousal Caregivers: How We Were Then, How We Are Now." *Psychology and Aging* 16 (2): 217–26.

Wilson, Kathi, Mark W. Rosenberg, and Sylvia Abonyi. 2011. "Aboriginal Peoples, Health and Healing Approaches: The Effects of Age and Place on Health." *Social Science and Medicine* 72 (3): 355–64.

CHAPTER 6

OLDEST AGE DOES NOT COME ALONE
"What's the Name of the Day?"

Mere Kēpa

SINCE THE NINETEENTH CENTURY, British settlement in Aotearoa, New Zealand, has drastically altered every aspect of Māori life, including care of *kaumātua* (older women and men). During pre-contact times, *whānau* (extended family) looked after their aged relatives, but this tradition has been disrupted, particularly in urban areas. The public health system that largely supplanted it was not designed with Māori in mind and has not necessarily served them well.

This chapter discusses a research project that investigated the situation and sought means to improve it. Titled "Bring Me beyond Vulnerability: Elderly Care of Māori, by Māori," it asked how Māori people could humanize the care *kuia* (older woman) and *koroua* (older man) received from the public system. It drew on traditional Māori principles to encourage an ideal of what a better, passionate system would be like. The chapter also reflects on my own experience as the primary, full-time, informal, and unpaid carer of my father, who had dementia for many years. I found that whānau-based care, in association with diverse people and organizations, could enhance the daily life of the parent with complex care, as well as the life of the exhausted, obligated carer. Indigenous peoples who are faced with changing societies and an aging parent will require an application in prayer. Thus, I offer the following prayer, *He whānau katoa* (We are all in this together).

"We" refers to the kuia or koroua, the carer, their families and friends, and organizations.

He whānau katoa. (We are all in this together.)

We offer you our hands
to do your work.
We offer you our feet
to go your way.
We offer you our eyes
to see as you do.
We offer you our tongues
to speak your words.
We offer you our minds
that you may think.
Above all, we offer you our hearts
that you may love;
we offer you wholesome care and love.

In New Zealand, the number of seniors (aged sixty-five and older) is rising, and those aged eighty-five or more are expected to increase from 1 percent to 6 percent of the total population by 2050. Māori constitute 14 percent of New Zealanders, but few reach the age of eighty-five; in fact, they make up less than 0.2 percent of the country's very old (Statistics New Zealand 2007). Those Māori who do reach the age of seventy-five commonly have multiple health problems, and due to their children's migration to urban areas, often for employment, whānau may not be available to take care of them. There is also a gender imbalance among the aged Māori seniors; that is, life expectancy for Māori males is seventy-nine years, whereas for Māori females it is eighty-six years. In addition, Māori people who reach advanced age (eighty plus years) tend to experience greater levels of frailty (Hayman et al. 2012). Although older Māori may enjoy wider social connections than non-Māori through their roles and responsibilities in their whānau and communities, their formal education is poor and their level of income is low. These facts are likely to affect their health and longevity (Hayman et al. 2012). Demographic projections predict that Māori will live longer than they do now, thereby expanding the numbers of senior Māori and accentuating the disparities in disability.

In 2008, Alzheimer's New Zealand estimated that 41,183 New Zealanders had dementia. Of these 1,483 (3.6 percent) were Māori (Martin and Paki 2012). Māori, being the largest group affected by dementia after European/other people, will require specific service and care practices that are grounded in their language and cultural values. To ensure that this occurs, whānau and *iwi* (tribe), the Christian church, friends, and families ought to perpetuate humanizing approaches to (memory) care before the next generation of very old Māori reach what should be a place of honour in their society, only to find that their position does not differ from that of the current generation.

He Whānau Katoa I Roto Tēnei Mahi: We Are All In This Together

Māori lived together as interconnecting groups within cultural, social, political, and economic systems that supported population survival and growth (Durie 2003; Dyall et al. 2014; M. Kēpa and C. Kēpa 2006; Salmond 1991). Their average life expectancy was similar to that of Europeans, approximately twenty-eight to thirty years (Pool 1991), but their lives were grounded in sound public health principles. For example, they had a system to provide clean water, to preserve and store food, to practise suitable hygiene and waste disposal, to separate the sick from the dead, and to draw on extensive local knowledge to produce medicines and remedies. Hence, before the advent of British colonization, Māori lived well in a wholesome and healthy environment.

However, this balance was upset during the nineteenth century, as increasing numbers of Europeans settled in New Zealand, expropriating Māori land in the process. By approximately 1860, they outnumbered Māori, becoming the dominant group in the country, normalizing the nuclear family, and espousing the values of individualism, competition, and consumerism. As a result, every aspect of Māori life was changed, including health and health care, typically not for the better. Since the mid-twentieth century, more and more Māori have been moving to urban centres, where they draw on the public health system for support if they know how to access the available services (Martin and Paki 2012). In rural areas, Māori who have any illness or disability, including dementia, are still cared for by whānau, often without any assistance from the public system. Unfortunately, fewer and fewer Māori remain in their rural communities on the *whenua* (land), close to or on their *marae* (sacred meeting place), with strong social, cultural, political, and spiritual connections to their whānau and whenua (see the glossary of Māori words at the end of this chapter).

In 2004, the research project titled "Bring Me beyond Vulnerability: Elderly Care of Māori, by Māori" set out to identify the vulnerability of

Māori in the New Zealand health system, and to determine how Māori could humanize their care. At that time, I was the project leader. We conducted interviews and focus groups with Māori seniors, their carers (informal, unpaid) and caregivers (formal, paid), and Māori health providers and community leaders in four New Zealand locales.

The Elderly Care project, as the study became known, focused on vulnerable Māori of sixty-five and older. The word "vulnerable," which entailed unequal power relations, was defined broadly to encompass people who could no longer care for themselves physically, emotionally, and legally. Some experienced diminished responsibility due to physical and mental illness; some were simply living alone in impoverished and isolated conditions, often too proud to succumb to being cared for; some were already institutionalized, even on a day care basis; some were living with whānau and had lost their financial independence, typically the government's universal pension.

The project's title expressed its position as a sociopolitical challenge to the notion of older Māori people's vulnerability that exists in Māori communities and in the prevailing English-speaking, European Pākehā society (M. Kēpa and C. Kēpa 2006). The title also indicated that the research was to be transforming and was to propose a humanizing practice of care that respected and used the reality, history, values, traditions, experiences, and imagination of Māori as integral parts of looking after older people within their whānau. Significantly, Sir Mason Durie (2003, 85) explains that a "reciprocal relationship exists in Māori society between kaumātua (older people) and community. A positive, if demanding, role is complemented by an assurance of care and respect." This relationship was encapsulated in a personal communication that was written by a kuia from Ōtaua in the north of New Zealand and sent to me by a research partner. She wrote, "He whānau katoa tātou i roto i tēnei mahi. We are all in this work together."

Admittedly, the public health system has attempted to develop positive relationships with and comfortable systems for older Māori, focusing on providing needs assessment techniques and service co-ordination to do so. Nonetheless, the development and focus do not preclude the need to involve Māori people themselves in improving the care of Māori seniors. Although it is sensible for Māori to draw on promising and useful aspects of the public system, whānau, iwi, and Christian organizations ought not to assume that automatic application of the right techniques and services guarantees successful care of Māori, especially those who rely solely on a government pension and are uneducated in the formal sense (Dyall et al. 2014).

In June 2005, the preliminary findings from the Elderly Care project were presented at the Hawaii Public Health Association Pacific Global Health Conference in Honolulu. A few months later, in November, the findings were presented at the fifty-eighth Annual Scientific Meeting of the Gerontological Society of America in Orlando, Florida. The project's final report was submitted in 2006 to the funder, Ngā Pae o te Māramatanga. In 2008, aspects of the study were published through New Zealand's education system, in the Māori language, for use by students in Te Kohanga Reo (Māori language nests), Te Kura Kaupapa Māori (Māori language primary schools), and Te Whare Kura (Māori language secondary schools). Local media networks also published aspects of the research. The researchers were invited to present to an audience of bilingual and bicultural kaumātua (leaders) residing in a rural area. Lastly, the project's Māori methodology, which informed a longitudinal study of successful aging, has been published by scholarly, Indigenous journals (M. Kēpa 2015; M. Kēpa et al. 2014).

"What's the Name of the Day?"

My personal connection with dementia predated the Elderly Care study by several years. For nearly a decade, I awoke listening for the sound of *tihei mauriora!* The "sneeze of life; life is good" signalled that my father had lived through another night. He died at the age of ninety years and ten days, on April 30, 2007. Six years later, I still hadn't shaken the habit of listening for the sound of my father breathing. There is comfort in the sanctity of the sneeze, in the belief that life is good because we feel people's love, just like we feel the warmth of the sun. No matter how small and unimportant my father and I are in the celestial context, the whānau understand that we were conscious beings and that we feel emotions. We feel happy and unhappy in the company of the whānau. We enjoy being joyful together, and we suffer deep and appalling pain together as Indigenous peoples within the dominant society.

During the years that I was my father's primary, full-time, unpaid carer, I was completing a doctoral degree in education at the University of Auckland. Of course, looking after him involved multiple relationships with many individuals and organizations, all of whom played their role in his care. Take, for example, people in his own and his late wife's families, his iwi health provider, the local Christian day care centre, and my friends and colleagues at the university.

In the rural, tribal village that was my father's home, people believe that there is nothing that is not created for a purpose. Everything has a point, so when my father and I returned to his home on our frequent visits from the city of Auckland and he asked, "What's the name of the day?" all of us, including visiting whānau and friends answered respectfully by naming the day. Even so, he repeated the question day after day, week after week, month after month, and year after year until his death. On reflection, I realize now that his question had a greater purpose; indeed, he was telling people that he could no longer remember the name of the day. In the beginning, no one recognized that his question was a call for help, and we responded quietly with, "Monday, Dad," "Friday, Robert," or "Sunday, old man." At first, our replies were patient, tender, and caring, but they became hasty and curt as the years wore on. Not one of us made the connection between the repetition and the fact that his memory was diminishing.

There were other signs as well. On some evenings, he would make up to sixty-seven phone calls to whānau living nearby; he forgot to take his daily medication; and he overlooked eating. Meanwhile, he never forgot to feed his dog and cats the best cuts of meat and fish brought to him by whānau and friends. He began to barricade the doors of his home – "digging in" – just as he had done during the Second World War when he was sergeant in the 28 Māori Battalion (A Company) attempting to protect his men from German gunfire in North Africa and Italy. He was no longer able to drive his beloved green Holden car to the local bar, where he would enjoy a "jug or two" and spin a yarn with his mates after a hard day's work on the farm. After his eightieth year, his distrust of the whānau and friends grew noticeable, and by his eighty-fourth year, my sister and I had become distressed by his behaviour.

Our father's health, culture, and social and political status were complex. He was a *rangatira* (chief), a kaumātua (leader), a soldier, and a best friend. Children like to think of their father as being brave and able to take care of anything and anyone. It did not occur to us that, one day, he would become very old and lose his memory. Eventually, we had to come to terms with the realization that he would never recover his faculties to lead our whānau again, and that a substantial part of taking care of him was to prepare him and ourselves for his death.

In pre-contact times, kaumātua like my father were the custodians of knowledge and traditions, which they meticulously taught to their whānau. Some of them cared for the children, teaching specific skills such as weaving, carving, and fishing, whereas others advised and counselled on combat. The role of the kaumātua entailed being Māori; guiding/leading; being strong, kind, and generous; and being wise in thought and deed. Their example in performing ceremonial duties, conducting protocol and greeting and hosting guests on marae, and resolving disputes meant belonging to the land and blood relations (Papakura 1986).

Children were seen as an integral part of whānau, and those who showed aptitude were selected and instructed in their interests by *pūkenga* (specialists). According to Richard Firth (1959), Joan Metge (1967), and Peter Buck (1970), young Māori men of *ariki* (aristocratic) status were instructed in the *wānanga* (a place of higher learning) to prepare them for leadership. Metge has written that the word "rangatira" has connotations of noble birth as well as chieftainship. The term has become a title that some Māori use to describe leaders outside their own areas. Metge also states that the title "kaumātua" is partly, not wholly, hereditary. Api Mahuika (1975) defines a kaumātua as a person who is a leader in Māori society, particularly on the marae. Ranginui Walker (1993) explains that a kaumātua is the leader of a whānau who makes decisions concerning the land shared by the extended family, the control and use of shared property, and the rearing and educating of children. The kaumātua was typically the recognized spokesman on the marae on behalf of the whānau. Roger Maaka (2003) clarifies that "kaumātua," which can be both a plural and a singular noun, is an inclusive word that applies to older men and women. The word not only defines an individual or a group as old but can also function as a title, much like "Elder" is used in Indigenous communities other than Māori. Durie (2003) notes that kaumātua play a significant role in connection with the *mana* (prestige, authority, control) of a whānau, keeping it flourishing beyond this life.

Colonization, assimilation, and urbanization have brought change to the status of both kaumātua and Māori society (Panapasa et al. 2013). In the twenty-first century, kaumātua have various social and political roles: they advise important figures both Māori and Pākehā; they sit on local council and university, school, and hospital boards; and they also play their essential linguistic and cultural role on rural and urban marae. As a kaumātua and a rangatira in his eighties and the sole surviving male of his siblings, our father had always been concerned with raising and educating children; protecting the integrity and prosperity of the whānau, the land, and the Māori language and culture; and launching an aggressive and sustained response to any outside forces that threatened them. In accordance with his status, he continued to attend whānau meetings, especially on the marae, sitting quietly, listening and conducting the ritual of ceremonial blessing in Te Reo Māori (Māori language) as required.

Memory Loss and Being Safe in Our Families' Arms

Old age rarely travels alone: memory loss is the close companion. Stories of this kuia or that koroua having behaved strangely in their oldest age abound among whānau, none of whom saw their actions as pathological. The kaumātua were simply becoming older, and they continued to live among whānau, at peace, until their temporary separation from us in death. No sense of danger, distress, fear, and disease prevailed among whānau. So why did all this change?

As mentioned already, colonization, assimilation, and urbanization altered the circumstances of kaumātua and Māori society. There is no assurance that any Māori deeply understands what happened to a way of living that was wholesome, more peaceful, less confusing, and not so expensive as the current one, and certainly not dominated by the health industry. Māori society and whānau are finding that unexpected memory loss has become a dangerous and distressing companion of old age.

But there is cause for optimism. Māori have a *pepehā* (tribal saying) that is instructive in understanding memory care, "Nau te rourou, naku te rourou, ka ora ai te iwi," meaning "With your basket and my basket, we will feed the people." The saying is about *utu* (reciprocity), a kind of act of love, of give and take. The saying informs whānau of ways of caring for the older relations. Even in his oldest days, my father would be guided by the saying; he would perform ceremonial duties on the marae in the countryside; he would greet and host guests in our home in the city; he would attempt to resolve disputes among our whānau, real and imagined. He believed simultaneously in *wairua* (spirits) and the Christian god. He imagined his ancestors, his late wife, and his mother – and he talked to them all. Every afternoon, at about four, he prepared our home like a fortress, ready for the German attack. He went to sleep late and slept fitfully. No sleeping pills for him, though. He maintained his work ethic, rising early to work on the land shared by his whānau in the tribal village, and he was guided by his late father until the last week of his life. In the city, every day, he attended the Christian day care centre near our home. He asked constantly for his mother, and he searched for his younger brother who was "blown to pieces" in the North African desert at the age of twenty-four, a victim of the Second World War. Once a kind father, a brave soldier, a rangatira, a kaumātua, and a loyal citizen of Māori society within New Zealand society, he was slowly and quietly becoming disturbed, confused, and distressed.

Māori people feel strongly about our freedom; we don't like being told what to do, as the dominant society has done for almost two hundred years. Our whānau didn't like being told by the doctor that father would die in two years if we removed him from his home in the country to our home in the city where he would be close to his sisters and nephews, the iwi health provider, the Christian day care centre, as well as the university. In fact, father lived seven more years. The health professional telling us that we should not take our father to his village, every month, was meaningless. Her advice that old Māori people would slowly lose the use of their first language was offensive and, of course, inaccurate. She was a health practitioner, not a linguist. Indeed, neither did we like the decontextualized lists of facts that were applied to father, nor the medicines prescribed to him without him knowing what was in them and how they would benefit him. And so, these are facts.

In truth, we like the feeling of comfort when doctors, consultants, and social workers are honest and offer coherent and cohesive information that supports whanau taking care of their parents. This comfort is grounded on the traditional Māori values of *whakapono* (trust), *aroha* (love), *manaakitanga* (care), *utu* (reciprocity), and *whanaungatanga* (harmony) (M. Kēpa and C. Kēpa 2006; M. Kēpa et al. 2014). Handed down from Māori antiquity, the principles influence the thoughts and conduct of the whānau in the present day. They are ancient and visionary, yet transforming, because they encourage an image of what a better health system and compassionate, wise nurses, doctors, directors, and managers would be like. They could also inspire Indigenous groups elsewhere, as well as people of an empirical bent in the broad area of health, and those who keep a finger on the pulse of governance and management.

Acting in concert, a whānau, an iwi health provider, a Christian day care centre, friends, and colleagues ought to perpetuate humanizing approaches to memory care that honour and respect Māori senior people, rather than treating them as a burden to the health system and society. Consequently, I finish by emphasizing that old age does not come alone. Seemingly insignificant questions such as "What's the name of the day?" may signal to whānau, to health providers, and to church organizations that something odd is happening to an older person. Undertaking more transparent research projects concerning memory loss and providing more compassionate memory care is imperative for vulnerable seniors in Māori society and other Indigenous societies. Research studies in successful aging and gerontology should make available clear information and the best technology and pharmaceuticals to the health professionals who look after octogenarians and nonagenarians experiencing memory loss. At the same time, compassionate care by whānau, carried out with the love and support of friends, colleagues, health organizations, and Christian day care centres, ought to be deeply infused with a spirit of duty, reciprocity, obligation, trust, generosity, knowledge, wisdom, and goodness. These are irrevocable facts.

Glossary

Aotearoa	The Māori name for the North Island, now applied to New Zealand itself
ariki	aristocrat, high status or rank
aroha	1. To love, feel pity, feel concern for, feel compassion, empathize; 2. Love, affection, sympathy, charity, compassion, empathy
He whānau katoa i roto tēnei mahi	We are all in this together
iwi	Extended kinship group, tribe, nation, people, nationality, race. Often refers to a large group of people descended from a common ancestor
kaitohutohu	adviser
kaumātua	older women and men
koroua	older man
kuia	older woman
mana	prestige, authority, control
manaakitanga	hospitality, kindness, care
manawa ora	hope
Māori	1. In this chapter, the word applies to the language and culture of the Indigenous peoples of Aotearoa, New Zealand. It is used interchangeably with Tangata Whenua; 2. Māori also means normal, usual, natural, common

marae	1. The sacred meeting place of whānau, iwi; 2. The courtyard – the open area in front of the Meeting House, where formal greetings and discussions take place. Often also used to include the complex of buildings around the marae
Mātauranga Māori	wisdom, knowledge
Mātauranga whakaaro	philosophy
Ngāti Pōrou	tribal group of East Coast area north of Gisborne to Tihirau
Pākehā	New Zealanders of European descent
pepehā	a tribal saying, proverb, formulaic expression, figure of speech, motto, or slogan
pūkenga	1. A lecturer, specialist; 2. A repository, expertise
rangatira	1. A chief (male or female), landowner; 2. The qualities of a leader are a concern for the integrity and prosperity of the people, the land, the language and other cultural treasures (e.g., oratory and song poetry), and an aggressive and sustained response to outside forces that may threaten these
Tāmaki-Ma-kau-rau	1. Auckland isthmus; 2. Auckland
Te Kohanga Reo	Māori language nests
Te Kura Kaupapa Māori	Māori language primary schools
Tihei mauri ora!	The sneeze of life, the call to claim the right to speak
utu	1. To repay, pay, make a response, avenge, reply; 2. Revenge, cost, price, wage, fee, payment, salary, reciprocity. An important concept concerned with the maintenance of balance and harmony in relationships between individuals and groups and order within Māori society, whether through gift exchange or as a result of hostilities between groups. It is closely linked to mana and includes reciprocation of kind deeds as well as revenge

wairua	Spirit, soul, quintessence – spirit of a person that exists beyond death
wānanga	a place of higher learning
whakapono	1. To believe; 2. Faith, creed, belief, trust
whānau	1. To be born, to give birth; 2. Extended family, family group, a familiar term of address to a number of people. In present-day society, it can include friends who may not be kin or blood relations
whanaungatanga	Relationship, kinship, sense of family connection. A relationship through shared experiences and working together, which provides people with a sense of belonging. Whanaungatanga is created as a result of kinship rights and obligations, which serve to strengthen each member of the kin group. Whanaungatanga also extends to others with whom one develops a close familial friendship or reciprocal relationship. Harmony
Whare Kura	Māori language secondary schools
whenua	land

Acknowledgments

Thanks to my extended families in northern and eastern Aotearoa, to my Tongan friends and their families in Aotearoa for their love and support of my care of my late father. I acknowledge the financial and preparatory support provided by Nga Pae o te Maramatanga and the LiLACS NZ team, School of Population Health, the University of Auckland.

References

Buck, Peter. 1970. *The Coming of the Maori*. Wellington: Whitcombe and Tombes.

Durie, Mason. 2003. *Ngā Kāhui Pou: Launching Māori*. Wellington: Huia Publishers.

Dyall, Lorna, et al. 2014. "Cultural and Social Factors and Quality of Life of Māori in Advanced Age: Te Puāwaitanga o Ngā Tapuwae Kia Ora Tonu – Life and Living in Advanced Age: A Cohort Study in New Zealand (LiLACS NZ)." *New Zealand Medical Journal* 127 (1393): 62–79.

Firth, Richard. 1959. *Economics of the New Zealand Maori*. Wellington: R.E. Owens.

Hayman, Karen J., et al. 2012. "Life and Living in Advanced Age: A Cohort Study in

New Zealand – Te Puāwaitanga o Ngā Tapuwae Kia Ora Tonu, LiLACS NZ: Study Protocol." *BioMed Central Geriatrics* 12: 33. DOI:10.1186/1471-2318-12-33.

Kēpa, Mere. 2015. "Partnership, Production and Exchange of Knowledges." *Journal of Indigenous Research* 4 (2015). http://digitalcommons.usu.edu/kicjir/vol4/iss2015/1.

Kēpa, Mere, and Corinthia Kēpa. 2006. "Bring Me beyond Vulnerability: Elderly Care of Māori, by Māori. Kei Hinga Au E, Kei Mate Au E. Te Tiaki a Te Māori I Te Hunga Kaumatua Māori." Final Report prepared for Ngā Pae o te Māramatanga/ New Zealand's Māori Centre of Research Excellence, hosted by the University of Auckland.

Kēpa, Mere, Corinthia A. Kēpa, Betty McPherson, Hone Kameta, Florence Kameta, Waiora Port, Hine Loughlin, Paea Smith, and Leiana Reynolds. 2014. "E Kore E Ngaro Nga Kakano I Ruia Mai I Rangiatea: The Language and Culture from Rangiatea Will Never Be Lost in Health and Ageing Research." *AlterNative* 10 (3): 266–87.

Maaka, Roger. 2003. "Perceptions, Conceptions and Realities: A Study of the Tribes in Maori Society in the Twentieth Century." PhD Thesis, University of Canterbury.

Mahuika, Api. 1975. "Leadership, Inherited and Achieved." In *Te Ao Hurihuri*, ed. M. King, 86–113. Auckland: Hicks Smith and Sons.

Martin, Ros, and Paea Paki. 2012. "Towards Inclusion: The Beginnings of a Bicultural Model of Dementia Care in Aotearoa New Zealand." *Dementia* 11 (4): 545–52. DOI:10.1177/1471301212437821.

Metge, Joan. 1967. *Rautahi: The Maoris of New Zealand*. London: Routledge and Kegan Paul.

Panapasa, Sela, Mere Kēpa, Waiora Port, Betty McPherson, Leiana Reynolds, Paea Smith, and Florence Kameta. 2013. "Optimal Aging and Evidence Based Research in Indigenous Populations, Te Kaumatuatanga: Indigenous Ageing in Advanced Age in Aotearoa, New Zealand." Paper presented at the Gerontological Society of America's sixty-sixth annual scientific meeting, New Orleans, November 20–23.

Papakura, Makareti. 1986. *The Old Time Maori*. Auckland: New Women's Press.

Pool, Ian. 1991. *Te Iwi Maori: A New Zealand Population, Past, Present, and Projected*. Auckland: Auckland University Press.

Salmond, Anne. 1991. *Two Worlds: First Meetings between Maori and Europeans, 1642– 1772*. Auckland: Viking.

Statistics New Zealand. 2007. *New Zealand's 65+ Population: A Statistical Volume*. Wellington: Statistics New Zealand. http://archive.stats.govt.nz/browse_for_stats/ people_and_communities/older_people/new-zealands-65-plus-population.aspx.

Walker, Ranginui. 1993. "A Paradigm of the Māori View of Reality." Paper presented at the David Nichol Seminar ix, Voyages and Beaches: Discovery of the Pacific 1700–1840, Auckland.

A FECUND FRONTIER
We Listen ... in between Talk ... We Listen

Jean E. Balestrery and
Sophie "Eqeelana Tungwenuk" Nothstine

>> What follows is a conversation between two women from different worlds.
Sophie is an Inupiaq Elder, originally from Cape Prince of Wales, a remote
village in rural Alaska, who now resides in Anchorage. Jean, of Euro-
American ancestry, is a member of the lesbian, gay, bisexual,
transgender, two-spirit, queer community, originally from the Lower 48,
or the contiguous United States, with childhood roots in São Paulo,
Brazil. They initially met in Nome, Alaska, in 2002 as social work
colleagues and forged a bond that has continued ever since. For these
women, the listening in between talk is an act of love. As Sophie
welcomes Jean to her Indigenous homeland, Jean welcomes
spaciousness in Euro-American contexts. The following conversation is a
fecund frontier, with relational messiness and respective histories
clashing in the present. Through many comings and goings, and gifts
reciprocated back and forth, these two women reveal resilient hearts. By
meeting in the middle – in the middle of different worlds and different
histories – they engage in mutuality, and in this engagement is the gift of
healing.

Beginnings ...

"To this day, I never greeted anyone like I greeted you when I first met you."

I listen

"I am Inupiaq from the village of Wales, Cape Prince of Wales, Alaska. Inupiaq means 'the real people.' I have a bachelor's in social work and three years of a master's in social work, but did not graduate. English is my second language since the day I was born. My thoughts and life experiences are only from me, other lives are not the same as mine."

Her name is Sophie, Sophie "Eqeelana Tungwenuk" Nothstine. She is an Alaska Native Inupiaq Elder from the village of Wales. We first met in Nome on a Monday – January 14, 2002. This was the first day of my new job: clinician on the Mobile Adolescent Treatment Team, in the Behavioral Health Services Department of Norton Sound Health Corporation. Based in Nome, this Alaska Native non-profit organization serves the Bering Strait region.

"I was an alcohol and drug abuse counsellor travelling with clinicians to the villages, helping out and bridging the gap between Native and non-Native."

I was born and raised in the village of Wales, and we all spoke my Native language, Inupiaq – every one of us in the village. And then I moved to Nome when I was nine or ten years old, and I was traumatized by the Western system ... I was made fun of for wearing my mukluks, kuspuk, and parkie because I dressed different than Western-system and English-speaking children, because I spoke my own Inupiaq language. Also, as I live internalized oppression, I live it every day – that's what you see with my people. My people have kept their hurting in for so long that they don't know how to say what they want without hurting other non-Native people."

>> The hub city of Nome lies in the Bering Strait region, which is inhabited by 9,492 people who are scattered across 45,000 square miles. About 75 percent of them are Native people. Nome itself has 3,598 residents, about half of whom are Native. Surrounding Nome are fifteen outlying villages, which comprise Native people. There are few roads outside of Nome, so travel is by plane, riverboats in summer, and snowmobiles in winter (Norton Sound Health Corporation 2014).

Real places are imbued with history and meaning, particularly among Indigenous peoples. As Thomas Thornton (2008, 4) explains, "for Tlingits, and perhaps all indigenous peoples, place is not only a cultural system but the cultural system on which all key cultural structures are built." A real place is a physical geographical context; it is "a framed space that is meaningful to a person or group over time" (Thornton 2008, 10). A connection to place can invoke a "culture of belonging" whereby one can "feel at home"; it is "a landscape of memory, thought and imagination" (hooks 2009, 221). An Inupiaq Elder describes this connection between place and belonging:

> There are few people in America who can say that their forebears were here ten thousand years ago. That is a powerful feeling. To know that your ancestors played with the same rocks, looked at the same mountains, paddled the same rivers, smelled the same campfire smoke, chased the same game, and camped at the same fork in the river gives you a sense of belonging that is indelible. (Hensley 2009, 18–19)

"We are still dealing with trauma from the Western system, from the United States government. It is genocide of my people. It takes five generations to wipe out a culture, and my grandkids' children are the fifth generation."

I listen

"I have difficulty bridging the gap between Western ways and Native traditional ways. We are lost. The next generation beneath me is lost, and the generation after that is also lost. As soon as the language dies off, there's no more culture."

Sophie shares with me some of her family pictures while talking about how she struggles to prevent cultural loss among her people.

"I was born and raised very traditional, mother and father and a brother and sisters, but when I moved away from our village and moved to Nome, I had nothing – no more comfort, personal comfort. Life was very traditional at Wales, where I was born and raised. I went to Nome, and that's when I got traumatized by this Western school system. Even though there were Native people there, I was looked down upon. It really did affect my esteem and self-worth."

I listen

"I helped start my village of Wales dance group – along with my son, Gregory Nothstine, and my nephew, Richard Atuk: the Kingikmuit Dance Group. We perform all over. Our traditional dancing is very spiritual for all Alaska Native peoples – Aleut, Inupiat, Tlingit, Tsimshian, Yupik, Athabascan – and drumming is the heartbeat. It's uplifting and powerful."

I listen

"The Elders are not speaking up, because the government system. We need to start listening. We need to help my generation. The white people may need to speak up to the government system first since they brought the white people here, but it's painful too,

*because even my own grandkids
don't always listen to me, or
show respect to me as an Elder
– the way I was taught by my
mom and dad and our Elders,
the way it used to be when I was
growing up, but I still try to teach
them."*

Sophie and I share many stories
with each other as we travel and
work together in the remote
villages near Nome. This job was
the most difficult and rewarding
experience of my life – truly, a
quintessential paradox!

*"Many non-Natives from the
Lower 48 come up here to hide,
and many are looking for their
spirituality because they have
lost it."*

I reflect upon the "non-Natives"
to whom Sophie refers. Many
people in Nome and surrounding
areas are indeed an eclectic
group of folks, striking me as
caricatures. There is the
adventurer – the outdoors person
who thrives living off the land,
and there's the recluse, the misfit
– I remember a comment made
by one of my housemates when I
lived in a large home near Front
Street: "Nome is the misfit capital
of the world!" There's also the
runaway, who hides or runs away
from something in the Lower 48,
as Sophie says, and yes, the
seeker too, who is looking for

something that is missing, or the companion to the seeker, the lost soul. All these types are easily identified. I wonder, as I reflect upon the lot of non-Natives in this most rural area of the United States – literally in the middle of nowhere – who am I?

>> As Gerald Mohatt and Lisa Thomas (2006, 95) explain, "Alaska Natives, though often viewed from outside Alaska as a single group, comprise over 225 federally recognized tribes that are also separate villages scattered throughout rural Alaska." Mohatt and Thomas list the major cultural groups, which have their own subsistence economies, cultural practices, and rituals: "in the north, the Inupiaq; in the interior, the Athabascan; in the southwest, the Yup'ik and Cup'ik; in the south and west along the coast and Aleutians, the Aleut and the Alutiiq; and to the southeast, the Tlingit, Haida, and Tsimshian."

"I have never seen a non-Native work with my people the way you do. You understand, because you and I are coming at the same issue but in different ways. You were helped being raised in part by your grandmother and when you were a little girl living in São Paulo, Brazil."

During my first year of living and working in Nome, I would often run to Front Street, "the edge of the world," as many call it, and jump across the larger-than-life boulders that mark the border between the street and eternity to run out onto the sea ice, singing and dancing as I listened to my Walkman and waving my arms all around. I imagined myself to be a bird, light as a feather, and snow falling sideways. I fell in love with nature's elements – and, yes, "the real people" too!

"You are real, not fake, that is why my people like you. White people don't trust each other, they don't say it like it is. You and I do, that's also what makes it difficult, maybe because it's hard to be real, afraid to be real 'cause one might fall apart at the seams."

The work with Sophie's peoples was extremely trying at times, particularly in the villages. "I don't need this!" I scream aloud as Sophie and I debrief our collaborative work back in the private space of the village-based counsellor's office. I share with Sophie: "I did not sign up to be treated this way, to be so disrespected by your people. The rudeness is unbearable."

I listen

I share with Sophie what I really think and feel: "I'm over it, Sophie! This is all for the birds! I'm outta here! I am not a martyr!"

I listen

>> Historical trauma is an organizing concept that describes the experience of distress among Indigenous people. For more than five hundred years since initial contact with Europeans, they have been subject to chronic trauma, dispossession, and displacement (see Brave Heart and DeBruyn 1998; Brave Heart-Jordan 1995; Duran and Duran 1995; Evans-Campbell 2008; Napolean 1996). Maria Brave Heart (2004, 9) notes that "forced assimilation and cumulative losses across generations, involving language, culture and spirituality, contributed to the breakdown of family kinship networks and social structures."

"My people are still suffering. When they see you, all they see is a white face and then they take it out on you, but you – just like every other non-Native who is here – didn't cause what happened to my people hundreds of years ago."

I listen

"We have, what is it? It's called something like 'historical trauma' – but it's still happening. It's the past in the present. You didn't cause it, so you shouldn't have to be so mistreated. I'm sorry, Jean. I know you are only trying to help."

Sophie hugs me. I cry, as she holds me in her arms. I feel her care, and as I do I begin to wipe the tears from my eyes. Once again, she gifts me with real understanding.

>> Specific to Indigenous peoples in Alaska, historical trauma encompasses the "Great Death," the influenza epidemic of 1900 that originated in

Nome and spread throughout the state, "killing up to 60 percent of the Eskimo and Athabascan people with the least exposure to the white man" (Napolean 1996, 10–11). There are three primary phases of historical trauma among Indigenous people in Alaska: "Introduction of Western illnesses and diseases, Western Education (Boarding Schools), and forced Western Christianity" (La Belle and Smith 2005, 1).

"There were entire villages that were wiped out in the early 1900s during the flu epidemic. A few people from my village went to Shishmaref but they couldn't get in because they quarantined it, and so that is why they did not get the flu. From 500 of Wales people, only 250 lived and few Elders and mostly adolescents, oldest twenty-one years, my dad was one of them."

Sophie cries and I watch her wipe the tears from her eyes with tissue. I feel my heart ache. I ask to hug her and she says "yes."

"Be quiet please. You are too loud, be quiet. You need to learn to be quiet and silent. You talk too much. I can't stand that with you." Jean talks so loud, and my Native people are taught to talk quiet. Silence is spiritual like the earth. Jean drives me nuts with her loudness too. We drive each other crazy but love each other.

These are the moments when I hit a wall. I am being myself, my jovial self (however loud!), and Sophie tells me to be quiet!

A Fecund Frontier **155**

Sometimes it is so frustrating to work with her, to be around her, that it literally drives me crazy! During some village trips, I honestly did not know if I would make it. During the tougher times, my telephone calls to debrief with my (non-Native) supervisor were what kept me in the game. Sophie told me that people who have worked with her before had difficulty working with her. Well, I know why: she can be so rude, abrasive, and bossy! What am I doing out here in the middle of nowhere anyway? And, no appreciation! What difference am I making – really?

"My parents never drank or smoked cigarettes. They were Christians, going to church every Sunday at First Methodist Church in Nome. They prayed before each meal and at bedtime, although my mom's mother and stepfather were drunks. I used to be one of those drunks on Front Street. Now I have forty-one years' recovery from alcohol abuse, since June 8, 1975, and before that I tried to commit suicide. Now, I take it one day at a time. One of my sons still won't talk to me. I have tried to talk with him, but he's not ready. He's been homeless and drinking every day and would

rather stay that way. I haven't
seen him since his sister Denise
King died in 2010. No one knows
where he is. My other son is
sober thirty years."

I listen

"So, when I snap at you, it's not
you, it's the trauma and my pain.
I'm one of the very few Elders that
will speak up because I am able
to speak up without falling apart.
I have had to go through years of
therapy, Alcoholics Anonymous,
and some re-evaluation
counselling, just to be where I
am. I've learned that since
childhood, because my sisters,
my mother, and father never
listened to me or heard me out, I
guess that's what I feel coming
from you, is that – what I felt from
my parents and my sisters – no
acknowledgment whatsoever,
that I'm not being understood or
being respected. It's the same
thing, I feel like I'm not heard.
Anyway, [crying] it just hurts, for
you and I both. I had seven sisters
and one brother, all from Wales,
and I'm next to youngest."

I share with Sophie about my
family of origin and my
childhood years: living in São
Paulo with my family – my
mother, father, and two brothers
– moving back to the States, and
my sister and other relatives who
live in Brazil.

A Fecund Frontier **157**

I listen

I share: "So, that is the reason I talk with my father nearly every day, Sophie, and why I get excited to call him. I am just getting to know him now, while I am up here in Alaska, because he just moved back to the States from São Paulo, and he lives with his only living relative – his brother in California."

"This is a very similar place. You are in the country but not in the United States. It is very similar here to what you experienced in Brazil."

In many ways, I feel "at home" here in this area of Nome and the villages. Why? Many reasons. When I first climbed Razorback Mountain in Sophie's home village of Wales, she said to me, "Enjoy your climb, but be careful. There is a gravesite up there. You will never forget this time in your life, you are a free spirit, and you will never experience the same freedom as you do here." As I sat atop Razorback Mountain, I drank in what I saw: the dark massive blue body of the Bering Sea that lost itself at the horizon, the dancing beams of light, the sun's rays across the waves, Big and Little Diomede Islands, and farther out the coastline of Russia. I swallowed the freshest of cool air, filling my lungs, transcending and holding the air in for as long as I could before gasping to finally let it out. I was still. I was silent. I was at peace. I could sit in that place for days.

I observe

While living and working in Nome, I reflected upon my larger goals and often wondered about whether I should pursue further schooling, a law degree? A doctorate in social work? Could I even do such a thing? Was I capable? I had many doubts.

Comings and Goings

"Think about getting your doctorate degree. You have potential, inner strength, and determination."

Sophie was the third Elder to encourage me to return to school for doctoral studies. She shared this support following similar encouragement I received from my father and a professor from my social work master's program.

>> In October 2004, Sophie treated me to dinner during the two weeks I was in Anchorage and en route to the Lower 48. She had recently moved back to Anchorage from Nome to reunite with her daughter and grandchildren. I was heading back to the Lower 48 to reunite with my own personal support system.

In the spring of 2008, I began pre-dissertation research in Alaska. On my travels out to Nome, Sophie accompanied me as an Elder cultural consultant. As we waited together in the Nome airport, she said, "Well, here we go again, hurry up and wait." We both laughed and laughed!

In summer 2009, we were invited to give a talk at an academic conference in the Lower 48, whose theme was on aging and Indigenous peoples. We arrived two days before our scheduled presentation.[1] We co-presented as a method of reciprocity, honouring our diverse perspectives.

I am thrilled to see Sophie again! I am moved and honoured that she made it, travelling twelve hours for this collaborative project. She says to me, "You wondered if I would make it, huh?" She knows me; she gets me. We arrive at our hotel, visit a little bit, and then get a good night's sleep.

"What! You don't have a PowerPoint done?"

"No. It will be okay."

"No, we need to do a PowerPoint! I'll call my son to get pictures."

I smile and chuckle. I remember when we worked together at a village called Koyuk, and Sophie taught the schoolchildren an Eskimo dance that had been dormant for fifty years. Back in Nome, we received an update from Koyuk's counsellor, who told us that some of the kids now came knocking on her door, asking to do the Eskimo dances

I listen

"There will be more challenges ahead, and I give you permission to choose the easier path."

"What does this mean?"

– an ineffable sweetness. I share with Sophie about my work in the doctoral program – about the challenges and opportunities, the costs and benefits associated with various paths for my dissertation.

I share: "Working with you and your people, it seems to be the path where my heart continues to return, even in the midst of all these challenges."

At the conference, Sophie and I are scheduled to speak first, at eight in the morning. On the evening before our talk, we discuss and revisit the questions that our conference mentor suggested we use for our co-presentation. We were supposed to get together with him, but the meeting has fallen through. We have not done this before: co-present in an academic conference setting.

For what seems like a couple of hours, I attempt to explain the questions for Sophie, and she has difficulty in understanding them. I get exhausted and essentially give up, telling her just to talk about whatever she wishes.

I am trying to understand. First, you don't help me and then you want to give up. I get so angry. Ahhhh! I raise my voice, throwing my arms in the air!

Yet, I feel as if she is not listening to me. I feel that I am in a no-win situation and I say: "I am not effectively explaining what these questions mean and you get upset; so then, I tell you to talk about whatever you want, and you still get upset. I suggest that we call Willa," a spiritual counsellor whom we have both consulted, and Sophie agrees. Willa helps us to manage our respective frustration and exhaustion. After about thirty minutes, Sophie and I get off the phone and agree that whatever is meant to be in the morning is meant to be. Not meeting with our mentor really threw us off.

"I agree. I am sorry, Jean, about getting angry at you. We will do just fine tomorrow. So long as we are together, everything will be okay."

"I am sorry for getting short with you too, Sophie. I'm just a little stressed. I've never done anything like this before, and I have no idea what to expect tomorrow."

>> On day one of the conference, Sophie and I are first to present. We are reminded that all speakers have about twenty minutes to give their talk, with five to ten more minutes for questions from the audience. Though I already knew about this timeframe, I feel conflicted in the moment as I am situated between two worlds: Sophie and her Native traditional world and the Western academic world. My heart aches.

Though I am hesitant, a bit uncomfortable in speaking before Sophie, who is an Elder, I nonetheless begin our co-presentation. I provide a context for our collaboration – a collaboration that began in social work practice and now continues in research. Then, Sophie walks to the podium and begins speaking.

"Well, Jean and I, we argued with one another for most of the day and evening yesterday, trying to get ready for today."

The audience laughs, and I smile as I look at Sophie. This is exactly what I love about her: she is real and honest; she unabashedly says what she thinks!

"We worked in the villages together. Jean has lived among my people. She helps with translating between our traditional ways and the Western system."

Sophie shares about her life history, experiences, and family as I manage the PowerPoint slides projected behind her.

"My father was a reindeer herder."

Sophie shares about her historical trauma and pain. She shares about our work together, past and present. Because she is an Elder, I ask for her permission to speak whenever I add to her comments and connect them to my paper.

>> Sophie's comfort and confidence visibly increase as she speaks, and at the twenty-minute mark she is warned to end her presentation. She acknowledges this yet continues speaking, only to be overtly cut off a few minutes later. Sophie then becomes discombobulated, but she acquiesces and we leave the podium, returning to our seats among the audience.

"Uh-oh, I guess here goes my career!" I think to myself. I can feel the tension in the room; it's palpable. Yet, Sophie smiles at me and wipes the back of her hand across her forehead while simultaneously puffing out a breath of air. We hug each other as we sit down. I smile and feel a calm rush over me. My heart expands.

"Look at the signs, they say 'Native Elder Conference,' but where are all the Native Elders? There are only two of us here."

"It is so painful, dealing with this Western system [crying]."

Sophie is astute. She observes.

I listen

"It is so shaming."

That evening, back at our hotel, Sophie and I debrief. "Thank you, Sophie. You were wonderful today, and I was honoured to be witness."

"Thank you, Jean. I am grateful for you in my life, and I hope I didn't ruin anything for you [hugs Jean]. Love you."

"Love you too," I say, as I wipe tears from my eyes. I don't remember when we began to acknowledge our love and deep regard for one another, it just sort of happened.

"Remember, I keep telling you, we are dealing with two different worlds: the ego and the spiritual, for eternity they shall never meet."

"Sometimes I tell you things to tell myself."

I listen

"Thank you, Sophie." I thank her from the depth of my heart for taking the time and effort to travel all the way from Anchorage to be with me at this conference.

"You have me and my family."

I tear up, receiving the gift of her welcome to me – more than that, her acceptance of me. In her presence, I always belong.

"I am here for you, always."

We are both salmon swimming upstream, and yet our bond has us building bridges from our respectively different places, driven by hope as we keep meeting in the middle.

>> On the second day of the conference, a Native researcher tells me, "Jean, we were talking this morning, and we knew better when Sophie got cut off during her presentation. We should have said something. We are sorry about that, and we need to apologize."

At the end of this morning's session, I watch researcher after researcher approach Sophie and give her a hug. I smile. I too receive hugs.

>> At the lunch break, our conference mentor asks if he can sit with us. Sophie says, "Sure." He apologizes for not having met with us before we gave our presentation, and Sophie immediately says, "I am disappointed." He avoids making eye contact with her and tells us that the other researchers were very impressed with our "cross-cultural collaboration." He explains that "it is the exact opposite of helicopter research and what we are all striving to work toward as a model – but we wonder how it could ever be replicated." Sophie responds, "Well, why not? We're doing it, aren't we?"

"It's painful to see my Native people like this, it's what you say, that word – colonizing. Yes, they have lost their Spirit. It is very sad and painful."

I listen

>> This conversation, between two women from different worlds, occurs within context of distinct ancestries. Sophie is of Indigenous ancestry

and Jean is of Euro-American ancestry. While these respective histories clash in the present, the listening in between talk is healing. Alison Jones and Kuni Jenkins (2008, 471) write that

> the juxtaposition of these stories does not simply enable multiple voices to speak; rather, it allows the indigene-colonizer relationship to be interrogated in uneasy ways that insist on examining power and common sense, as well as the place of histories in the present. In this tension is the fecundity of collaboration.

"Hi, Sophie." Since I began my doctoral program, not a week goes by that I do not talk with Sophie, and there are long periods of time when I talk with her daily. I have hit many walls during my studies.

I listen

She talks me through.

"You are a survivor and you can do it. I'm proud of you. You are doing the impossible. I know you are fighting for your life, and I'm proud of you for it. Well, did you think it was going to be easy? If it were easy, everyone would be doing what you are doing."

I gasp for air in between the oceans of tears that I cry. "Thank you, Sophie, for all your support, I know you understand. I don't think I could be doing this without your support. Love you."

"I always knew you could do it, and you have double whammy:

social work and anthropology
too! You are doing good work. It
must be difficult because you are
doing things differently. I always
knew you would do good work."

I listen

>> As Jean and Sophie listen in between talk, each learns more about the other's lived experience. As each learns more about the other's lived experience, the heart strengthens. As the heart strengthens, mutual acknowledgment deepens. Linda Smith (2008, 117) states,

> I would emphasize the importance of retaining the connections between the academy of researchers, the diverse indigenous communities, and the larger political struggle of decolonization because the disconnection of that relationship reinforces the colonial approach to education as divisive and destructive. This is not to suggest that such a relationship is, has been, or ever will be harmonious and idyllic; rather, it suggests that the connections, for all their turbulence, offer the best possibility for a transformative agenda.

"Truth is a function of power." This comment was made by a professor in one of my classes, referring to a journal article we read. Yet, reflecting upon the experience of the conference where Sophie and I co-presented, I realized the paradox of this notion "is also just as real: Power is a function of truth" (Balestrery 2014, 266).

"The ego and the spiritual shall never meet."

I listen

I hold up my two hands, bringing them close together, palm to palm, almost touching yet not.

I watch

〉〉 In 2011–12, we are working together in Alaska. We travel from Anchorage to Nome, to Sophie's home village of Wales, and then to the neighbouring village of Shishmaref.

"I love your village, Sophie!"

"Why's that?"

"Well, first, because it's your village, and I love visiting your relatives, but I also think it's the most beautiful village! I love Razorback Mountain and I love the freedom I feel there. It's the farthest point west in the United States – so we are literally at the edge of the country!"

I laugh

I laugh too. I adore Sophie's laughter. It is infectious. When she laughs, the world around her laughs – it's true!

〉〉 Sophie shared with Jean about her deep connection to the land, describing it as cultural: "My people are of the earth." Keith Basso (1996, xiii) asks,

What do people make of places? The question is as old as people and places themselves, as old as human attachments to portions of the earth. As old, perhaps, as the idea of home, of "our territory" as opposed to "their territory," of entire regions and local landscapes where groups of men and women have invested themselves (their thoughts, their values, their collective sensibilities) and to which they feel they belong. The question is as old as a strong sense of place – and the answer, if there is one, is every bit as complex.

It's September 2012, and the thirteenth annual Kingikmuit Dance Festival is upon us. I am welcomed as a visitor to Wales and see many people whom I have known for over a decade, including residents and visitors from Nome and other villages.

"Sophie! I was asked to dance, and so I did!"

"Good for her."

At first, I don't know what Sophie means by "her," but then I realize that she's talking about her relative, the woman who asked me to dance. She's happy because her relative is becoming accepting of me as a "white face" …

"My people don't want to see a white face in the villages."

I listen, and I follow. In the villages, I am a visitor.

"I am so confused."

"How come?" I ask, as I prepare morning coffee in the village of Shishmaref.

"I have relatives in this village and they haven't come to visit me yet. When we worked together before in the villages, my relatives would always come visit me wherever I am."

"You're right, I remember. What do you want to do?"

"I guess we can go visit them at their house."

"Sure."

"Jean, these are my relatives."

Sophie introduces me to an Elder and his wife.

"Lots of changes in the village, huh, since we were all growing up together."

I listen

>> In the summer of 2013, Sophie and I are invited to share about our work – about how we collaborate across lines of difference – at an Indigenous research gathering in Canada.[2] Beforehand, I travel from the Lower 48 back to Anchorage for another fieldwork follow-up visit.

"Sure, of course I want to go, but we aren't doing dementia research?"

"I know, but we are working in the area of indigeneity. I explain further."

I listen

"Does that make sense?"

"Yep, now I understand. We are doing things differently, and there are people – Native and non-Native alike – who will go against us."

*"I only do what the lord above
tells me to do. I am only human."*

Travelling together takes a lot of
preparation and patience. It is a
process of struggling and
surrendering, a going back and
forth, a juxtaposition of forces
– forces that I initiate and also
forces to which I respond. We are
both human.

"Why not you?"

I laugh and laugh.

"Why me, Sophie?"

I smile and I laugh.

I could have done a much easier
project, you know. This has been
challenge after challenge – in
the system and the community.

*"Yep, and do you think this has
been easy for me? [laughing]
Heck no! Sometimes we both go
kicking and screaming, but you
are hanging in there – I don't
know how you do it."*

*"You are doing well. I'm amazed
at how well you are doing."*

"Well, sometimes, I don't know
either."

"I don't know how you do it
either, you are hanging in there
too! Love you!"

"Love you too!"

It is the first day of the research
gathering, and we co-present in
the afternoon. I ask Sophie if she
would like to begin, and she
says, "No, go ahead." So I lead
at this time, and Sophie follows.

"What did she say?"

"I'm raging inside."

"Sounds good. Let's go."

"Okay, Jean, will you please help me walk down there?"

I walk to the podium in the centre of the floor, and she sits in a chair beside me. I begin by acknowledging the kuspuk I am wearing as a gift from Sophie – a gift for me to wear today.

I repeat to Sophie what another researcher in the audience just said as commentary about our collaboration. She said she can see the love between us and it's beautiful. And then Sophie responds to this researcher –

I am silent, while the audience chuckles. Sophie does not want her own or her people's pain to be lost on others even though she is smiling. Together, we are real. "Sophie, it's time now to go to the evening session, which is the community panel and where you are one of the invited speakers."

We gather again at the roundtable. All the invited panel speakers are asked to walk down to the centre table.

"Sure." I hold out my arm for Sophie to take as she walks down the aisle stairs. Sometimes she uses her cane, and sometimes she doesn't. We arrive at the table, and I ask her if she wants me to stay sitting beside her.

"Yes, please."

I hesitate, as this is *her* time, but then again, I want to respond to her wishes. So, I find another chair to sit in, and I position it beside yet behind both her and the other speakers at the table.

"I think what is happening here is really great. When I was growing up, I never heard about this dementia. We didn't have a word for it in my Inupiaq language. It's a problem, though, so we need to deal with it, but just like with everything else, we need to do it slowly, otherwise, it will be retraumatizing".

Tears keep rolling down my cheeks as I listen to Sophie speak, and speak. The last time we attended an academic conference, she was cut off. This time, I am prepared to support Sophie and her voice, but to my amazement, nobody cuts her off. I keep wiping away tears as I listen, and listen, bearing deep witness.

"Quyanna."

>> As bell hooks (2000, 164) writes, "a generous heart is always open, always ready to receive our going and coming. In the midst of such love we need never fear abandonment. This is the most precious gift true love offers – the experience of knowing we always belong."

*"You come from your culture, I
come from my culture, and we
meet in the middle."*

I listen

>> Ours is a relationship of resilient hearts. Over the years, we have had
many comings and goings across diverse places and spaces. It is messy,
for sure, but we both keep meeting in the middle.

"Welcome home!"

I reciprocate. "Love you, Sophie!
Quyanna!"

Love you too, Jean! Quyanna!

Talk with Sophie is talk with a
touchstone.

... We listen ...

... in between talk ...

... We listen ...

Concluding Here, Yet Continuing On ...

Although this chapter has reached its end, the journey continues. At one
point, Jean asked Sophie, "Do you think what we are doing is going to
help at all?" Sophie replied, "Oh yes, it will. If it helps even just one
person, it has all been worth it."

Acknowledgments

This research was supported by grants from the John A. Hartford Foundation,
the RUTH LANDES MEMORIAL RESEARCH FUND, a program of
the Reed Foundation and the University of Michigan School of Social Work
and Department of Anthropology, including the National Institute on Aging
Training Grant (T32-AG000117). We would like to thank all the reviewers,

including Wendy Hulko and Danielle Wilson, research assistants Anna Parkscott and Jessica Gates, and Natahnee Nuay, for providing helpful feedback on earlier drafts.

Notes

1   Importantly, Jean secured funding to cover all the expenses for both herself and Sophie to attend the conference. This is congruent with recommendations in Indigenous literature, whereby Indigenous community collaborators do not incur financial burden from participation in research.

2   Our expenses were covered by the hosts at this gathering, so there was no financial burden upon either of us.

References

Balestrery, Jean. 2014. "A Multi-sited Ethnographic Study in Alaska: Examining the Culture-Communication Nexus Salient to Alaska Native Elders and Conventional Health and Social Services." PhD diss., University of Michigan.

Basso, Keith H. 1996. *Wisdom Sits in Places: Language and Landscape among the Western Apache.* Albuquerque: University of New Mexico Press.

Brave Heart, Maria Yellow Horse. 2004. "The Historical Trauma Response among Natives and Its Relationship to Substance Abuse: A Lakota Illustration." In *Healing and Mental Health for Native Americans: Speaking in Red*, ed. Ethan Nebelkopf and Mary Philips, 7–18. New York: Altamira Press.

Brave Heart, Maria Yellow Horse, and Lemyra DeBruyn. 1998. "The American Indian Holocaust: Healing Unresolved Grief." *American Indian and Alaska Native Mental Health Research* 8 (2): 56–78.

Brave Heart-Jordan, Maria Yellow Horse. 1995. "The Return to the Sacred Path: Healing from Historical Trauma and Historical Unresolved Grief among the Lakota." PhD diss., Smith College.

Duran, Eduardo, and Bonnie Duran. 1995. *Native American Postcolonial Psychology.* Albany: State University of New York Press.

Evans-Campbell, Teresa. 2008. "Historical Trauma in American Indian/Native Alaska Communities: A Multilevel Framework for Exploring Impacts on Individuals, Families and Communities." *Journal of Interpersonal Violence* 23 (3): 316–38.

Hensley, William L. Iggiagruk. 2009. *Fifty Miles from Tomorrow: A Memoir of Alaska and the Real People.* New York: Picador.

hooks, bell. 2000. *All about Love: New Visions.* New York: HarperCollins.

–. 2009. *Belonging: A Culture of Place.* New York: Routledge.

Jones, Alison, and Kuni Jenkins. 2008. "Rethinking Collaboration: Working the Indigene-Colonizer Hyphen." In *Handbook of Critical and Indigenous Methodologies*, ed. Norman K. Denzin, Yvonna S. Lincoln, and Linda T. Smith, 471–85. Thousand Oaks, CA: Sage.

La Belle, Jim, and Stacy Smith. 2005. "Boarding School: Historical Trauma among Alaska's Native People." Prepared for the National Resource Center for American Indian, Alaska Native, and Native Hawaiian Elders, University of Alaska, Anchorage.

Mohatt, Gerald V., and Lisa R. Thomas. 2006. "'I Wonder, Why Would You Do It That Way?' Ethical Dilemmas in Doing Participatory Research with Alaska Native Communities." In *The Handbook of Ethical Research with Ethnocultural Populations and Communities*, ed. Joseph E. Trimble and Celia B. Fisher, 93–115. Thousand Oaks, CA: Sage.

Napolean, Harold. 1996. *Yuuyaraq: The Way of the Human Being*. Fairbanks: Alaska Native Knowledge Network.

Norton Sound Health Corporation. 2014. "Life in Bering Strait Region." https://www.nortonsoundhealth.org/careers/life-in-bering-strait-region/.

Smith, Linda T. 2008. "On Tricky Ground: Researching the Native in the Age of Uncertainty." In *The Landscape of Qualitative Research*, ed. Norman K. Denzin and Yvonna S. Lincoln, 113–43. Thousand Oaks, CA: Sage.

Thornton, Thomas F. 2008. *Being and Place among the Tlingit*. Seattle: University of Washington Press.

PART 3

APPLYING THEORY AND KNOWLEDGE TO PRACTICE

CHAPTER 7

DEPRESSION, DIABETES, AND DEMENTIA

Historical, Biocultural, and Generational Factors among American Indian and Alaska Native Elders

Linda D. Carson, J. Neil Henderson, and Kama King

DIABETES AMONG AMERICAN INDIANS and Alaska Natives, as well as in other Indigenous populations, constitutes a glaring health disparity when compared with the prevalence of diabetes in non-Indigenous populations. Factors shared by Indigenous and other colonized populations include prolonged generational exposure to enormously high levels of physical and emotional stressors, which intertwine with biomedical and cultural factors to contribute substantially to disease states. In this chapter, the causal connections between depression, diabetes, and dementia are examined. We discuss historical, biocultural, and generational factors that may contribute to the high prevalence of dementia in diabetic American Indian and Alaska Native (AI/AN) elders,[1] and present a biocultural perspective of diabetes, depression, and dementia.

The Biocultural Model of Diabetes, Depression, and Dementia

The biocultural perspective, or "Biocultural Model," as termed by Ann McElroy (1990), combines biological and cultural factors in one of two ways: "segmented," in which the factors that contribute to disease states are seen as linear and discrete variables, sequentially ordered; or "integrative," in which all the factors interact, influencing outcomes in either positive or negative ways. In his Chronicities of Modernity Theory, Dennis Wiedman (2012) uses McElroy's integrative model in examining the ways in which diabetes, culture, and centuries-long stressors become enmeshed to worsen the burden of disease in American Indian populations. (For an extensive discussion of various additional models, see Chapter 2 in this volume.)

The construction of clinical realities is made up of intricate interactions between social practices, biology, and cultural frames of meaning that are passed down through generations (Kleinman 1980). Research suggests that one possible source for the persistent and increasing prevalence of diabetes among Indigenous and other enslaved peoples is deeply embedded psycho-cultural factors. These may perpetuate a cascade, from the advent of depression due to life events, intergenerational traumatic memory, and nutrition trauma to the development of diabetes, a notable risk factor for stroke and subsequent vascular dementia.

The Physiology of Oppression

"Physiology of oppression" refers to the physical outcome of prolonged stress under extremely prejudicial and traumatic conditions (Scheder 2006). It is experienced by formerly colonized and/or enslaved people and can be recognized in American Indians, Alaska Natives, African Americans, and Indigenous populations worldwide. Colonialism, enslavement, cultural stress, structural violence, intergenerational traumatic memory, nutrition trauma, and contemporary trauma: the outcome is the physiology of oppression.

Life under forced colonization and structural violence is characterized by emotional and cultural trauma. Traumatic memories of past events are handed down through the generations, affecting the physical and emotional health of populations that suffered abuse on multiple levels. These memories may revolve around systematic enslavement, involuntary assimilation, discrimination, racism, impoverishment, and culture loss. During the process of forced assimilation, children were removed from their families and often placed in boarding schools. Relocation practices such as the Trail of Tears, instigated by the US Congress through the passage of the Indian Removal Act of 1830, resulted in the death of over half the American Indian population during its removal to other states. Dwelling sites were extremely disrupted and destroyed. Populations were removed from and denied access to their traditional burial grounds, where souls, life, and death are thought to reside (Henderson et al. 2010).

Subsistence patterns were destroyed by neocolonialism when access to hunting and foraging was denied through compulsory relocation to poor land that was barely able to sustain life. Physical activity was restricted through internment on these arid lands. Population density increased as multiple tribal groups were transported into ever-smaller areas. Food supplies dwindled. Tribal populations experienced what has been termed "nutrition trauma" (Korn and Ryser 2006).

Remember that for all peoples, food practices are imbued with cultural meaning and constitute more than simply "nutrition." Food is part of cultural life. Traditional celebrations and rites of passage, which bring families together, typically involve food sharing and perpetuate the culture and solidify cultural ties. Relocation ended access to traditional food sources, and the food provided to the colonialized groups was lacking in nutritive value and was sometimes spoiled. As Mary Peters, an Oglala Sioux from Spirit Lake, recalled, "We once ate the right foods and lived the right way as *Wakan Tanka* intended us to do. People used to live to a very old age, before we were put onto reservations" (Lang 2006, 64).

There is contemporary trauma as well. Institutionalized discrimination and racism exist within the social service system, with the result that needed services are difficult to access and sometimes denied. Over time, Congress has steadily decreased the funding for medical care that is offered though the Indian Health Service. The Indian Health Service meets less than 50 percent of primary care needs. Congress has also systematically decimated the Department of Agriculture food programs, such as the commodity foods and food stamp programs.

Biocultural Mechanism of Action

The amalgam of biocultural factors that leads to the physiology of oppression begins historically with colonialism and possible enslavement of population groups for various political, economic, and sociocultural reasons. The acquisition of land, racial prejudice, war, and fear of unknown Indigenous peoples are just a few of the motivating factors. For colonialized people, the result is intergenerational traumatic stress and traumatic memory. A Yurok elder noted that "Indian people have always been watched and controlled," and an Oglala elder, referring to diabetes, stated, "It is worry that brought it on, all the stress we have now" (Lang 2006, 64).

In American Indian tribes, there is a sense that diabetes is caused by the white man and by being forced to eat the white man's diet. For example, in a study of Oklahoma Choctaw elders with diabetes, a participant commented, "If it wasn't for the white people, we wouldn't have all these problems. Traditional cooking is good, white cooking is bad. The wild game is gone (due to whites)" (Henderson 2002, 84).

Linda Carson Henderson (2009) discusses the belief among Oklahoma Choctaw elders that life events and stress are directly correlated with the development of diabetes. Stress alone causes neuroendocrine patterns of emotional response. The fight-or-flight response, in which the autonomic nervous system produces additional oxygen and nutrient supplies, including glucose, causes the secretion of cortisol. This leads to the breakdown of carbohydrates, proteins, and lipids. In stress-free times, insulin acts through the hypothalamus (which has both hunger and satiety centres) to decrease food intake and body weight. When an individual is chronically stressed, however, cortisol acts on cells throughout the body, making them insulin resistant. At the same time, the body releases the high levels of glucose that are needed to combat stressors. Overly high levels of cortisol stimulate the appetite, especially sugar cravings, and weight gain (Mendenhall 2012). Figure 7.1 illustrates the complexity of these interactions.

FIGURE 7.1 Interactional biocultural model of diabetes, dementia, and depression

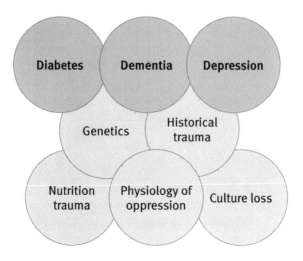

Depression

When diabetes is first diagnosed, the shock of diagnosis and resultant depression may adversely affect both an individual's ability to self-manage the condition and his or her motivation to seek help from health care providers (Baldridge 2013; Fisher 2014). Emotional trauma or chronic stress (which itself may precipitate a major depressive disorder) are both associated with unstable blood glucose levels. This instability may actually precipitate diabetes in someone with normal glucose levels or may worsen existing diabetes.

The lifetime prevalence of depressive disorders in the United States ranges from 5 to 17 percent. Indeed, depression is a major cause of disability worldwide. However, despite the high prevalence, studies show that physicians in the United States fail to recognize the signs and symptoms of depression in 30 to 50 percent of depressed patients (Haber 2013, 60–62). Only 10 percent receive adequate treatment (Holroyd and Clayton 2000). One study conducted by Paula Trief (2007), which analyzed 389 videotapes of physician-patient interactions, found that assessments for depression occurred in only 14 percent of visits. The failure to recognize depression and to treat patients or refer them for mental health care has well-known far-reaching effects, including thoughts of suicide and exacerbation of co-morbidities, such as diabetes and cardiovascular disease.

The etiology and risk factors of depression are multifactorial, adding to the difficulty of prevention and assessment of depression. Family history, life experiences, the existence of chronic disease, and the environment all play interactional roles. In older adults, depression may arise from age-related changes in the brain and body. For example, cardiovascular disease, with concomitant stroke, may result in neurological damage. If this occurs, the older adult who has no family history of depression may develop what health care providers refer to as "vascular depression." Symptoms may manifest in the early stage of Alzheimer's disease before dementia occurs (NIH Senior Health 2013).

Further, the excessive levels of stressors that can lead to a depressive state may contribute to the development of diabetes. Diabetes is more common among Indigenous people than among other groups, and it is plausible that their historical and nutrition traumas, leading to their marginalized place in society, contribute heavily to their stress (Ferreira and Lang 2006). Therefore, the stressors may result in depression, which may then be a risk factor for diabetes. The high levels of stress-related cortisol mobilize glucose stores in the bloodstream, increasing the chances that a person will become diabetic.

The connection between depression and diabetes was recognized as early as 2008. A study by researchers at Johns Hopkins University hypothesized that there was a bi-directional association between depression and type 2 diabetes (Golden et al. 2008). The study included non-Hispanic white, African American, Hispanic, and Chinese individuals who were participants in the Multi-Ethnic Study of Atherosclerosis, a longitudinal cohort initiative. Findings suggested that persons with elevated depressive symptoms had an increased risk of developing type 2 diabetes, independent of other risk factors such as an unhealthy lifestyle. The research also found that individuals who were being treated for diabetes, but who had no symptoms of depression at baseline, were at significantly higher odds of becoming depressed during the follow-up period (Golden et al. 2008). Some researchers refer to this phenomenon as "diabetes distress" (Fisher 2014). Depression among diabetics quite often remains undiagnosed, and if it is diagnosed, it tends not to be incorporated into diabetes care plans (Baldridge 2013). According to the National Institute of Mental Health (NIMH 2011), "some symptoms of depression may reduce overall physical and mental health, not only increasing your risk for diabetes, but making diabetes symptoms worse ... Fatigue or feelings of worthlessness may cause you to ignore a special diet or medication plan needed to control your diabetes, worsening your diabetes symptoms."

The Diabetes and Aging Study (2004–10) was one of the first cohort studies to examine depression, Alzheimer's disease, senile dementia, presenile dementia, and vascular dementia in diabetes patients. It found that depression did indeed increase the risk of dementia in patients with type 2 diabetes. For these patients, depression was heavily associated with risk factors for the development of vascular dementia, such as poor adherence to diet and exercise programs, increased smoking, and ineffective blood glucose control. The research also identified psychobiologic changes in the subjects who had depressive symptoms. These changes boosted cortisol levels, thus increasing blood glucose levels, as described previously. In 2012, the Diabetes and Aging Study, having followed 3,766 patients with both depression and diabetes for a three- to five-year period, found that those with co-morbid depression had a 100-percent increased risk of dementia (adjusted hazard ratio: 2.02; 95 percent confidence interval: 1.73–2.35). Depression in diabetic patients was most definitely associated with an increased risk of developing dementia, as compared to those patients who were not depressed (Katon et al. 2012).

Diabetes Mellitus (Type 2 Diabetes)

Type 2 diabetes is a worldwide health issue whose prevalence is so great that researchers have begun to view it as pandemic. Table 7.1 compares its prevalence rate among American Indians/Alaska Natives (AI/AN) with that of other groups.

TABLE 7.1 Race and ethnic differences in prevalence rates of diabetes

Race/ethnicity	Percentage of population	Prevalence rate
AI/AN	14.2	142 per 1,000
Non-Hispanic whites	7.1	71 per 1,000
Asian Americans	8.4	84 per 1,000
Non-Hispanic blacks	12.6	126 per 1,000
Cubans	7.6	76 per 1,000
Mexican Americans	13.3	133 per 1,000
Puerto Ricans	13.8	138 per 1,000

SOURCE: Centers for Disease Control and Prevention (2011).

According to the Indian Health Service, 16.3 percent of AI/AN have diagnosed diabetes, and 30.0 percent of them have pre–type 2 diabetes (Indian Health Service 2011). The US Department of Health and Human Services gives the slightly lower rate of 14.2 percent. Additional data indicate that AI/AN may be as much as 2.2 times more likely than non-Hispanic whites to be diabetic. Those who have type 2 diabetes are 4.0 times more likely than their white counterparts to have an amputation as a complication. They are 6.0 times more likely to experience end-stage renal disease (Indian Health Service Division of Diabetes Treatment and Prevention 2012).

The commonly cited risk factors for type 2 diabetes (not in order of proportional contribution to variance) include metabolic syndrome, AI/AN ancestry, genetic factors (identified and unidentified), family history, being female, stress, history of gestational diabetes, obesity due to suboptimal nutrition, sedentary lifestyle, and depression.

Diabetes was not highly prevalent among AI/AN until approximately fifty years ago (1964). Sadly, their mortality rate from type 2 diabetes has increased 93 percent during the last twenty years (1994–2014). Even this is deemed an underestimation because more than half of all diabetic patients die of cardiovascular disease. Therefore, cardiovascular disease is often cited as the primary cause of death. Additionally, it has been estimated that fully 30 percent of AI/AN have pre-diabetes (Indian Health Service 2011). It should be noted that prevalence rates vary widely across tribal populations, so the true burden of diabetes is specific to each group. Population numbers can vary from tribe to tribe, and this too may add to the variance (see Table 7.2).

TABLE 7.2 American Indian and Alaska Native diabetes prevalence rates

Tribe/region	Percentage of population	Prevalence rate
Southern US tribes	26.7	267 per 1,000
Arizona tribes	33.5	335 per 1,000
Pima	>60.0	>600 per 1,000
Alaska Natives	5.5	55 per 1,000
Average	30.1	314 per 1,000

SOURCE: Centers for Disease Control and Prevention (2011); Indian Health Service Division of Diabetes Treatment and Prevention (2012).

Complications from Diabetes

The numerous complications of diabetes are well documented. They include end-stage renal disease; gestational diabetes (superimposed upon pre-existing diabetes), which can increase the incidence of diabetes among the children born to mothers with the condition; diabetic retinopathy (sometimes leading to blindness); neuropathy, which can entail peripheral vascular disease and amputation; and cardiovascular disease, including hypertension and stroke.

Diabetes contributes heavily to the risk of developing cardiovascular disease, with attendant hypertension, the outcome of which may be small strokes called transient ischemic attacks. If frequent, these may cause vascular dementia. Thus, the cause of vascular dementia among Indigenous populations is multifactorial. Examining modifiable risk factors for the development of this form of dementia is mandatory for health care providers and includes prevention and the instigation of early treatment for pre-diabetes, diabetes, and depression.

Depression, Diabetes, and Dementia   **187**

Dementia

The Indian Health Service has traditionally not collected statistical data on dementia. One unfortunate reason for this is that AI/AN elders did not survive to the age of greatest risk. At this time, statistical data concerning dementia prevalence and mortality are not available from the Indian Health Service's Department of Program Statistics. In any case, using death certificates to assess mortality rates may not be helpful, as patients with dementia may have multiple co-morbidities, making it difficult to pinpoint the exact cause of death.

Prompted by prior research with patients who had type 2 diabetes, which showed that their risk of developing dementia was twice that of the general population, the Diabetes and Aging Study, cited previously, assessed dementia rates. Its objective was to explore ethnic/racial differences in risk for dementia among those who had type 2 diabetes and those who did not. The study population consisted of 22,171 diabetic patients who were sixty or older. The data indicated that the age-adjusted dementia incidence densities were highest among Native Americans (34/1,000 person-years) and African Americans (27/1,000 person-years), as compared to non-Hispanic whites, Latinos, and Asians (Mayeda et al. 2014). Table 7.3 presents racial and ethnic differences in dementia and diabetes co-morbidity rates.

In Western Australia, a retrospective study was conducted on survival outcomes in dementia patients with and without diabetes. The results showed that the onset of dementia as well as death occurred an average of 2.2 and 2.6 years earlier, respectively, in subjects who had diabetes. In addition, there was an important correlation between age of onset for diabetes and that for dementia. Subjects who had been diagnosed with dementia before the age of sixty-five and who had been diagnosed with diabetes fifteen or more years prior to the diagnosis of dementia died almost twice as quickly as those who did not have diabetes (hazard ratio: 1.9; 95 percent confidence interval: 1.3, 2.9). Therefore, the study concluded that mortality from dementia and attendant co-morbidities was highest for people who developed diabetes before middle age (Zilkens et al. 2013).

Summary: Elders and Historical Trauma

When we examine the social determinants of health in regard to AI/AN, Indigenous, and other colonized peoples, it is apparent that many elders among them (defined by the Indian Health Service as those aged fifty-five and older) experience "multiple jeopardy." They are often politically

TABLE 7.3 Racial and ethnic differences in dementia and diabetes co-morbidity
rates

Race/ethnicity	Percent of study population	Prevalence rate
Prevalence of dementia and type 2 diabetes co-morbidity in patients diagnosed with dementia from Kaiser Permanente Northern California Diabetes Registry		
American Indians	19.0	190 per 1,000
African Americans	19.1	191 per 1,000
Latinos	15.0	150 per 1,000
Asian Americans	12.5	125 per 1,000
Non-Hispanic whites	17.8	178 per 1,000
Prevalence of dementia alone in total population by race and/or ethnicity		
Australians	6.5	65 per 1,000
Cree	4.2	42 per 1,000
African Americans	7.0	70 per 1,000
Non-Hispanic whites	7.2	72 per 1,000
Japanese Americans	7.6	76 per 1,000
Hispanics	4.2	42 per 1,000

SOURCE: Manly and Mayeux (2004).

disenfranchised, either presently or historically, are commonly poverty-stricken, and are in poor health, compared to their counterparts in the general population (Henderson 2002, 2010; Sokolovsky 2009). It is these older individuals who are at greatest risk for developing type 2 diabetes (American Diabetes Association 2018). If we look at these elders as the descendants of a long history of structural violence at the hands of colonizing nation-states, the concept of multiple jeopardy expands exponentially. Indigenous governments and scholars attribute the dramatically high chronic disease morbidity and mortality, as compared to that of the mainstream population, to structural violence, with its associated social and physical suffering, traumatic memory, community destruction, and nutrition trauma (Ferreira and Lang 2006; Korn and Ryser 2006; Roubideaux and Acton 2001). Health care for American Indians was previously administered by the Bureau of Indian Affairs, but it should be noted that the bureau once fell under the auspices of the secretary of war. Because studies of Indian health status showed such extensive morbidity and mortality, the Indian health program was transferred from the bureau to the Public Health Service in 1954 (Rhoades and Rhoades 2000).

We present the following words from an elder treated in the Bureau of Indian Affairs system as an example:

> I went to get my tonsils out at (an Indian Health Service hospital). I only got put part to sleep. The nurse came and got me. I stayed for two weeks to guard against bleeding. I also stayed at the hospital weeks before having a baby. My first husband ran off; he was "noholo" (white man; literal translation: person without a soul). I had to stay one month due to complications. There was a German doctor who told me when I was in pain that horses and cows don't have anything for their pain so I got no anesthesia. I tore badly. He was an awful man. The same one who took out my tonsils. (Henderson 2010, 312)

Clearly, the history of Indigenous interactions with the white community is an extremely important variable. Elders and their descendants are repositories of memories from times past, both from their own experience and that of their ancestors. The history of contact with whites is one of extermination ("the only good Indian is a dead Indian"), expulsion from lands, exclusion from mainstream society through internment on reservations, and attempted forced assimilation, including the removal of children to boarding schools (Holmes and Holmes 1995). In the traditional culture, there is considerable distrust of white persons, which is passed down as intergenerational traumatic memory. This has influenced numerous cohorts, causing an all-encompassing environment of stressors, which contribute substantially to the development of multiple co-morbidities.

The distrust of white authority is also evident in the AI/AN experience of tribal health care systems. Physicians, nurses, nurse practitioners, and physicians' assistants are sometimes seen as symbols of white authority, even if they themselves are AI/AN. In some instances, the distrust may prompt an AI/AN patient to listen politely as a health professional gives medical instructions but to subsequently ignore or even deride the advice upon returning home. Linda Carson Henderson (2002, 2009, 2010) found that obeying the directions of a health care provider could alienate elders from their peer group. One subject refused to take her diabetes medicine because she felt that the doctors were experimenting on her.

Implications

Health care providers must remember that the risk of depression increases in people who have been diagnosed with diabetes but must also note that the relationship between depression and diabetes can be bi-directional (Golden et al. 2008). This would mandate early recognition and treatment of depressive symptoms in seniors who have not been diagnosed with type 2 diabetes. Providers should also be aware that depression in older adults may have an atypical presentation (sometimes referred to as "masked depression"), difficult to assess. It is estimated that only about 10 percent of depressed elder individuals receive treatment. Therefore, practitioners should consider routine screening for depression among this group, just as they might routinely screen for diabetes and hypertension. The Geriatric Depression Scale is most useful here. Its short form could be used in clinical settings (Holroyd and Clayton 2000).

In the United States, health care providers to AI/AN, in collaboration with the Centers for Disease Control and Prevention, recommend several key steps for patients with possible concurrent diabetes and depression: educate patients about these conditions, screen all diabetics for depression, use multidisciplinary teams, and intensify case management for persons with depression (Indian Health Service 2011).

Perhaps future research and interventions might also assess the efficacy of modifying risk factors for depression that are associated with life under stressful conditions, as a strategy for facilitating diabetes prevention, education, treatment, and self-management. In populations that have suffered multiple political-economic and sociocultural traumas over the years, this becomes even more important. The social determinants of health linked to past histories of impoverishment and trauma play a considerable role in any clinical assessment, yet they are often ignored.

❖ ❖ ❖

The triad of depression, diabetes, and dementia must be examined within the amalgam of contributing biocultural factors, as depicted in Figure 7.1. Historical trauma, culture loss, ongoing nutrition trauma, the physiology of oppression, and genetic factors interact to produce the extremely high prevalence of type 2 diabetes in AI/AN, as well as in other Indigenous and colonized peoples. In addition to inadequate assessment and consideration of depression as a contributing factor, some strategies for diabetes prevention, education, and self-management may not be effective for AI/AN people. This may arise from the failure to understand the true etiology of type 2 diabetes and the multiple interacting biocultural factors in populations that experience health disparities. Identifying modifiable risk factors is an important step, but their elimination or mitigation in the AI/AN population may require assessment and strategies that differ from those used for mainstream, non-impoverished groups. Communication between care providers and Indigenous people should take into full consideration the long-standing nature of the contributing variables. Failure to do so may result in multiple co-morbidities, with tragic endpoints, such as vascular dementia due to cardiovascular disease, poorly controlled hypertension, and stroke.

History cannot be changed, but it can be recontextualized as an incentive to employ culturally relevant stress-reducing strategies, to recognize and acknowledge the true nature of historical trauma, and to diagnose depression early. Because depression interacts with multiple factors to precipitate type 2 diabetes, its early diagnosis and treatment may have a positive influence on the prevalence of diabetes over time. Adequate treatment for depression among diabetics will improve the self-management of their condition. With maximal control of both depression and type 2 diabetes, we can hope to avoid vascular dementia as an outcome, with its profound effect on families and tribal services.

Acknowledgments

We are grateful to the National Institutes of Health's National Institute on Minority Health and Health Disparities, as well as to David J. Baldridge, executive director of the International Association for Indigenous Aging.

Note

1   In this chapter, we follow the US Indian Health Service in defining an elder as a person who is fifty-five and older.

References

American Diabetes Association. 2018. "Statistics about Diabetes." http://www.diabetes.org/diabetes-basics/statistics/.

Baldridge, D. 2013. "Diabetes and Depression among American Indian and Alaska Native Elders." Atlanta: Centers for Disease Control Healthy Aging Program.

Centers for Disease Control and Prevention. 2011. "National Diabetes Fact Sheet:

National Estimates and General Information on Diabetes and Prediabetes in the United States, 2011." Atlanta: US Department of Health and Human Services. https://www.cdc.gov/diabetes/pubs/pdf/ndfs_2011.pdf.

Ferreira, M.L., and G.C. Lang. 2006. "Introduction: Deconstructing Diabetes." In *Indigenous Peoples and Diabetes,* ed. M. Ferreira and G. Lang, 3–27. Durham, NC: Carolina Academic Press.

Fisher, L. 2014. "Diabetes, Distress, and Depression." Centers for Disease Control National Center for Chronic Disease Prevention, Division of Diabetes Translation. https://www2c.cdc.gov/podcasts/media/pdf/DiabetesStressAnd-Depression Webinar.pdf.

Golden, S.H., M. Lazo, M. Carnethon, A.G. Bertoni, P.J. Schreiner, A.V. Diez Roux, H.B. Lee, and C. Lyketsos. 2008. "Examining a Bidirectional Association between Depressive Symptoms and Diabetes." *Journal of the American Medical Association* 299 (23): 2751–59.

Haber, David. 2013. "Clinical Preventive Services." In *Health Promotion and Aging: Practical Applications for Health Professionals,* 6th ed., ed. David Haber, 37–71. New York: Springer.

Henderson, J.N., L. Carson Henderson, R. Blanton, and S. Gomez. 2010, November. "Autopsy, Diabetic Amputations, and End-of-Life Issues among Elderly American Indian People." Paper presented at the American Anthropological Association annual meeting, New Orleans.

Henderson, L. Carson. 2002. "The Cultural Construction of Diabetes Mellitus among Oklahoma Choctaw Elders and Choctaw Nation Tribal Health Care Providers: An Examination of Concordance between Models and Implications for Care-Seeking and Compliance." PhD Diss., University of South Florida.

–. 2009. "Battling a New Epidemic: American Indian Elders and DM." In *The Cultural Context of Aging: Worldwide Perspective,* 3rd ed., ed. J. Sokolovsky, 550–67. Westport, CT: Praeger.

–. 2010. "Divergent Models of Diabetes among American Indian Elders." *Journal of Cross-Cultural Gerontology* 25 (4): 303–16.

Holmes, E.R., and L.D. Holmes. 1995. *Other Cultures, Elder Years.* Thousand Oaks: Sage.

Holroyd, M., and A. Clayton. 2000. "Measuring Depression in the Elderly: Which Scale Is Best?" *Medscape General Medicine* 2 (4).

Indian Health Service. 2011. "Indian Health Diabetes Best Practice: Depression Care." http://www.ihs.gov/MedicalPrograms/Diabetes/HomeDocs/Tools/BestPractices/2011_BP_DepressionCare_508c.pdf.

Indian Health Service Division of Diabetes Treatment and Prevention. 2012. "Diabetes in American Indians and Alaska Natives: Facts at-a-Glance." https://www.ihs.gov/MedicalPrograms/Diabetes/HomeDocs/Resources/FactSheets/Fact_sheet_AIAN_508c.pdf.

Katon, Wayne, Courtney R. Lyles, Melissa M. Parker, Andrew J. Karter, Elbert S. Huang, and Rachel A. Whitmer. 2012. "Association of Depression with an Increased Risk of Dementia in Patients with Type 2 Diabetes: The Diabetes and Aging Study." *Archives of General Psychiatry* 69 (4): 410–17.

Kleinman, Arthur. 1980. *Patients and Healers in the Context of Culture.* Berkeley: University of California Press.

Korn, Leslie E., and Rudolph C. Ryser. 2006. "Burying the Umbilicus: Nutrition Trauma, Diabetes, and Traditional Medicine in Rural West Mexico." In *Indigenous Peoples and Diabetes,* ed. Mariana Leal Ferreira and Gretchen Chesley Lang, 231–78. Durham, NC: Carolina Academic Press.

Lang, G. 2006. "'In Their Tellings': Dakota Narratives about History and the Body." In *Indigenous Peoples and Diabetes,* ed. Mariana Leal Ferreira and Gretchen Chesley Lang, 53–71. Durham, NC: Carolina Academic Press.

Manly, Jennifer J., and Richard Mayeux. 2004. "Ethnic Differences in Dementia and Alzheimer's Disease." In *Critical Perspectives on Racial and Ethnic Differences in Health in Late Life,* ed. Norman B. Anderson, Rodolfo A. Bulatao, and Barney Cohen, 95–141. Washington, DC: National Academies Press. https://www.ncbi.nlm.nih.gov/books/NBK25535/.

Mayeda, Elizabeth R., Andrew J. Karter, Elbert S. Huang, Howard H. Moffet, Mary N. Haan, and Rachel A. Whitmer. 2014. "Racial/Ethnic Differences in Dementia Risk among Older Type 2 Diabetic Patients: The Diabetes and Aging Study." *Diabetes Care* 37: 1009–15.

McElroy, Ann. 1990. "Biocultural Models in Studies of Human Health and Adaptation." *Medical Anthropology Quarterly* 4 (3): 243–65.

Mendenhall, E. 2012. "Narrative to Mechanism: Understanding Distress and Diabetes." In *Syndemic Suffering: Social Distress, Depression, and Diabetes among Mexican Immigrant Women,* ed. E. Mendenhall, 93–106. Walnut Creek, CA: Left Coast Press.

NIH Senior Health. 2013. "Depression: Causes and Risk Factors." https://www.nia.nih.gov/health/depression-and-older-adults.

NIMH (National Institute of Mental Health). 2011. *Depression and Diabetes.* NIH Publication No. 11-5003. Bethesda, MD: NIMH.

Rhoades, E., and D. Rhoades. 2000. "Traditional Indian and Modern Western Medicine." In *American Indian Health: Innovations in Care, Promotion, and Policy,* ed. E. Rhoades, 401–17. Baltimore: Johns Hopkins University Press.

Roubideaux, Yvette, and Kelly Acton. 2001. "Diabetes in American Indians." In *Promises to Keep: Public Health Policy for American Indians and Alaska Natives in the 21st Century,* ed. Mim Dixon and Yvette Roubideaux, 193–208. Washington, DC: American Public Health Association.

Scheder, Jo C. 2006. "The Spirit's Cell: Reflections on Diabetes and Political Meaning." In *Indigenous Peoples and Diabetes,* ed. Mariana Leal Ferreira and Gretchen Chesley Lang, 335–56. Durham, NC: Carolina Academic Press.

Sokolovsky, J. 2009. "The Ethnic Dimension in Aging: Culture, Context and Creativity." In *The Cultural Context of Aging: Worldwide Perspective,* 3rd ed., ed. Jay Sokolovsky, 277–87. Westport, CT: Praeger.

Trief, Paula M. 2007. "Depression in Elderly Diabetes Patients." *Diabetes Spectrum* 20: 71–75.

Wiedman, Dennis. 2012. "Native American Embodiment of the Chronicities of Modernity: Reservation Food, Diabetes, and the Metabolic Syndrome among the Kiowa, Comanche, and Apache." *Medical Anthropology Quarterly* 26 (4): 595–613.

Zilkens, R., W.A. Davis, K. Spilsbury, J.B. Semmens, and D.G. Bruce. 2013. "Earlier Age of Dementia Onset and Shorter Survival Times in Dementia Patients with Diabetes." *American Journal of Epidemiology* 177 (11): 1246–54.

CHAPTER 8

ADAPTING CIRCA-BC
in the Post-Residential-School Era

Barbara Purves and Wendy Hulko

MEMORY – ITS PRESERVATION AND LOSS – holds a special meaning for First Nations Elders. It can be shared through storytelling and passing on traditional knowledge, or it can be suppressed, as in the painful memories associated with residential schools. During recent years, however, the latter have been stirred up. In April 2008, the prime minister of Canada officially apologized for Indian residential schools, and two years later, the Truth and Reconciliation Commission (TRC) began its hearings, which ran from April 2010 to March 2014. It published its final report a year later (TRC 2015). Given this context, First Nations' views about memory and reminiscence as central concepts in dementia and dementia care may be different from Eurocentric biomedical views. With this understanding, we sought to explore the views of First Nation Elders on the customization of a software program for supporting reminiscence-based conversations with older British Columbians living with dementia, including those with Indigenous ancestry.[1] This exploration was part of a larger study (Purves et al. 2015).

Indigenous Views on Memory Loss and Dementia

Studies conducted by the contributors to this book and other researchers have revealed the variable meanings that Indigenous peoples attach to memory loss and dementia in later life. Qualitative studies spanning at least fifteen years determined that Indigenous families and communities did not have a good understanding of dementia or necessarily see it as problematic (see Garvey et al. 2011; Henderson 2002; Hulko and Stern 2009; Sutherland

2007). The word itself was not known or used in Indigenous groups (Hendrix and Swift Cloud-Lebeau 2006; Pollitt 1997). In fact, it has been suggested that dementia may be viewed in a positive light if symptoms are seen as communication with the spiritual realm (Henderson and Henderson 2002) and/or as enabling connections to one's ancestry (O'Connor, Phinney, and Hulko 2010).

Recent research in British Columbia with Secwepemc Elders (Hulko et al. 2010), in Saskatchewan with Cree grandmothers (Lanting et al. 2011), and in Ontario with Ojibwa, Oji-Cree, Cree, and Haudenosaunee Elders, healers, and community members (Jacklin, Warry, and Pace 2012) found that their understandings of memory loss and dementia are complex and nuanced in differing ways. Nonetheless, there are similarities. For example, the participants used the medicine wheel or the circle of life as a way of understanding and situating memory loss in later life, as in returning "back to the baby stage" (Lanting et al. 2011), "going through the full circle of life" (Hulko et al. 2010), or "coming full circle" (Jacklin, Warry, and Pace 2012), all of which signal a return to the spiritual realm. Despite these similarities, each group's understandings of the causes, risks, and prevention for dementia are sufficiently unique to caution researchers against pan-indigenizing, particularly in connection with culturally safe memory care.

Reminiscence in Dementia Care

Reminiscence has long been recognized as an effective way to promote social interaction with people who have dementia (Kim et al. 2006). They tend to retain memories formed in childhood and early adulthood, which can be stimulated by photos or other objects to provide a context for conversations (Fromholt and Larsen 1992). During such exchanges, people with dementia can sometimes recount stories about their past, which, even if fragmented, can give carers valuable insights into their unique history and personhood (Fels and Astell 2011).

The CIRCA program, or the Computer Interactive Reminiscence and Conversation Aid as it is officially known, was developed to capitalize on this (Alm et al. 2004). It uses touch-screen technology to allow users (normally a person with dementia and a conversation partner) to select photos, short film clips, or music to talk about together. These media are organized in several categories (such as entertainment, sports, and recreation), three of which are randomly selected each time users start up the program; subsets of items in each category are also randomly accessed in every start-up.

Research findings suggest that random access and touch-screen technology generate more equal participation between conversation partners, contributing to the program's effectiveness (Astell et al. 2010).

The original CIRCA program, which was first used in Dundee, Scotland, featured several hundred media items drawn from public archives. Because its intent was to stimulate long-term autobiographical memories of older people with dementia, its designers chose media that dated from the participants' youth in Dundee during the 1940s and 1950s. To explore the use of CIRCA in British Columbia, therefore, our first step was to select media from local public archives, also from the 1940s and 1950s, that would be familiar to long-time residents of the province. In undertaking this, we also explored strategies to best accommodate the diversity of BC communities and regions, including First Nations.

Knowing that images can evoke profound emotional reactions – both positive and negative – and being aware that attendance at a BC residential school was typically a traumatic experience, we felt it important to seek Elders' guidance in developing CIRCA-BC. Thus, we posed two research questions. First, images of First Nations people in the public archives from the 1940s and 1950s tend to reflect perspectives of colonization (Walsh 2008), so we sought guidance on how to represent First Nations people in CIRCA-BC. What kind of media should we include, and what images should we leave out? Second, we explored Elders' thoughts about using the program in their communities, especially given the research discussed above, which suggests that Indigenous understandings of memory loss and dementia may differ significantly from Eurocentric biomedically influenced views.

How We Sought Elders' Guidance

Our overall study (Purves et al. 2015) included focus groups to explore the perspectives of older adults on developing a CIRCA-BC program. The focus group described in this chapter consisted of First Nations Elders, all of whom lived near a small resource-based city in British Columbia. We received research approval from all appropriate university and health authority behavioural ethics boards. As the study was not conducted in partnership with a specific First Nation or community, we did not go through a separate approval process. However, we did observe protocol in other ways, including the provision of an honorarium to the Elder participants, gifting tobacco at the start of our work together, beginning each focus group session with a prayer, and taking a minimally directive approach to facilitation.

Participants

To recruit participants for this focus group, Wendy Hulko asked Elders whom she already knew from previous work with them about dementia. Four Elders from two nations agreed to participate. They completed a questionnaire that asked where they were born, where they had spent their lives, and which areas of British Columbia were familiar to them. The four Elders, who ranged in age from sixty-seven to seventy-eight, were born in British Columbia and had spent most, or all, of their lives there. All had lived in several regions of the province, and two had also lived in other provinces and/or the United States for extended periods.

Focus Group Procedures

The four Elders met for two sessions, each lasting approximately two and a half hours, which were conducted by Wendy Hulko or Barbara Purves and a research assistant. In the first session, following introductions, a welcome, and an overview of the project, including a description of the CIRCA-BC program, we asked for Elders' views regarding two broad issues. We had acquired photos, music, and film clips from local and provincial museums, university special collections, and archives of the Canadian Broadcasting Corporation, all of which dated from the 1940s to the 1960s and portrayed First Nations people in some way. We asked the Elders for their opinions on this material and whether they would include each item in the proposed CIRCA-BC program. We also invited them to suggest additional topics, such as people, places, events, or things that might prompt older adults to talk about growing up in the area. Second, we asked for their views regarding how (or if) the CIRCA-BC program could contribute to memory care for First Nations older adults. We also asked how to represent residential schools or if they should be included at all.

Guided by participant comments from the first session, we returned to the public archives to locate additional media. Then we held the second session, whose purpose was to solicit participant feedback about these new media and to revisit topics from the first session in light of them. Media presented in this session were not all specific to First Nations people and included some that had been found for other focus groups with participants from the same region. Both sessions were audio-recorded and transcribed.

We checked the transcripts and corrected them where needed. Next, we undertook a constant comparative analysis involving an iterative refinement of concepts and categories across the two transcripts to identify themes that emerged from the data. These were subsequently grouped into topics, drawing on Mark Luborsky's (1994) definitions and procedures for the identification of themes and topics. Following Luborsky's guidelines, we defined topics as broad areas of concern that are often (though not always) closely linked to researchers' questions. Themes, on the other hand, represent "the manifest generalized statements by informants about beliefs, attitudes, values, or sentiments" (Luborsky 1994, 195).

What We Learned

Our analysis of the sessions revealed several themes that, though overlapping and intersecting, could be broadly grouped into five topics, each of which addressed either our first question about the representation of First Nations in CIRCA-BC or our second question about how to use the program (if at all) with First Nations seniors, or both. Identifying topics provides a way of organizing the data, but the description of themes within each topic highlights the values, perspectives, and beliefs of the Elders.

The first topic, "memory and memory loss," which includes Elders' views about individual and collective memory, and about potential causes of memory loss, deals with both of our research questions. The second topic, "who we are," addresses themes that arose from participant discussion of being First Nations and of what contributes to that sense of identity; it is primarily relevant to our first question. "Residential schools," the third topic, is interwoven with the preceding two, but it alone specifically addresses the impact of colonization; it is relevant to both research questions. "What and how old people remember," the fourth topic, addresses participant views on the process of reminiscing and on images that could prompt it, as well as describing themes arising from their own reminiscences during the sessions. The final topic, "adapting CIRCA-BC for First Nations seniors," describes participant views about the program itself as a tool for supporting reminiscence.

Memory and Memory Loss: "Lights Went Out"

Elders raised the topic of memory and memory loss in several contexts. Sometimes, they linked it to dementia: "a lot of the Native people – some of the memory losses are dementia [and] are recent" (FG 1, 789).[2] However, memory loss was more often connected with the impact of colonization, affecting both collective and individual memory.

Elders associated collective memory with the intergenerational tradition of storytelling: "the types of teaching – one of them was, like, storytelling – and little kids sat by the Elders and listened carefully because everything, every story they told, was important" (FG 2, 285–87).

Another added, "everything that people knew in those days, before the Indian school days, it was passed down, passed down, passed down" (FG 1, 467–68). In this context, memory loss was seen as a consequence of colonization. One Elder linked it to a Secwepemctsín word meaning "lights went out."[3] He explained, "I think that part of the memory loss is that, the loss of your culture and language and things like that, and a lot of that stuff was forced" (FG 1, 37–39). Forced memory loss as the suppression of language and culture was a theme that recurred frequently throughout both sessions, with another participant commenting, "for me the lights went out when I was told not to speak my language, and getting hit when I spoke my language" (FG 1, 960–61). Collective memory too was overshadowed by forced history lessons: "They've been taking our kids to school and teaching them about *other* heroes that were building colonies and being imperial" (FG 1, 433–36). This speaker concluded, "the memories are for five hundred years, are not even our own" (FG 1, 444–45).

Collective memory loss was also associated with other consequences of colonization that disrupted the tradition of storytelling and intergenerational sharing of knowledge. These consequences included alcoholism, as one Elder explained:

> Everybody was drinking. And all the grandmothers stopped telling us stories, and all the grandfathers stopped telling the stories, or even the old people taking us up into the mountains to go medicine hunting and berry picking ... That was our life until the fifties, and then *all* of that disappeared. So, for me, it wasn't just healing residential school, it was healing the advent of drugs and alcohol. (FG 1, 1017–23)

Another Elder noted that diseases could result in the loss of shared stories: "One of the memory losses is when the diseases came through ... killed all of our stories and the Elders got killed, most of the Elders at the time" (FG 1, 1444–47).

Individual memory loss was also seen as a result of colonization. As one Elder put it, "some people choose not to remember. Like all of the residential schools and some of the traumas they went through, you know" (FG 1, 43–44). He went on to link this with his own life: "It was a big, big blank in my lifetime – right from six years old, when they took me, and right up until my thirties, I don't hardly remember anything because I didn't want to" (FG 1, 46–48). Elders also talked about the importance of healing as a necessary step to recalling any good memories. One stated, "My brain is healing up, and my body's healing, and some of the stories I was told before I went to residential school I'm starting to remember" (FG 2, 326–27). Another said that she was unable to recall any good memories associated with residential school "until after I healed all the trauma around getting beaten up" (FG 1, 1159–60).

In summary, in contrast to dementia, which Elders described as relatively recent and uncommon in their communities, memory loss emerged as multifaceted and pervasive. At the same time, they acknowledged the intertwining of the two, as shown in this remark: "hopefully what we've said has helped you understand a little bit more about whether it is dementia or whether it is senility, or whether it is people from those Indian schools that just don't want to remember. They want to erase that whole era" (FG 2, 507–9).

Who We Are: "Coming Home"

Several themes were interwoven within this topic. Elders discussed many of the values they associated with being First Nations and described aspects of everyday life that contribute to their sense of identity. Some comments alluded to an individual's sense of identity, whereas others referred to a local community or "our people," as in, "I found a picture of our people that had the long ones [headdresses]" (FG 1, 1442–43). However, a sense of shared identity with other First Nation cultures was also a strong theme. For example, an Elder mentioned being one of only three First Nations women who worked in a hospital: "*three,* out of what, five or six hundred people that worked there" (FG 2, 397–98). She added, "it was so wonderful to have somebody else that was part of your world – even though we came from all over Canada, we were part of that world that we came from" (FG 2, 399–401).

A second theme was the strong link between identity and place. Sometimes this was referenced by personal ties: "we were having a meeting up by that big golf course by the river ... and I pointed out where my great-great-grandparents used to park their horses" (FG 1, 57–60). It was also evident as Elders introduced themselves, when they described their connections to their family and their territory. For instance, after explaining that he had not attended residential school, one participant added,

> That's who I am. I grew up and we were still semi-nomadic right up till I was eighteen years old, I guess. Course, I didn't go with my mom and dad once I became fifteen, sixteen, and that. But I still went sometimes to the fishing grounds, and I know where they're all at, and berry picking, picking berries. I still retain a lot of that. (FG 1, 235–39)

A third theme was the importance of language for identity. During both focus group sessions, two Elders sometimes switched to Secwepemctsín. One stated, "I always try to use the language because I think that's part of the memory loss" (FG 1, 37–38). The other Secwepemctsín speaker also linked language and identity, this time in terms of humour, explaining that a great deal of the humour expressed in Secwepemctsín was "lost in translation" because English could not capture Secwepemctsín speakers' understandings of "what's funny and what isn't funny, what's real and what isn't real" (FG 2, 1866–68).

Interwoven with the themes of identity were themes regarding the challenge of living within the dominant culture. This included talk about colonizing efforts to suppress First Nations people and about resistance against such suppression. One Elder brought up the example of *lahal*, which is a traditional First Nations guessing game that involves two teams seeking to win from each other game pieces made of bone or antler. Traditionally, drumming and singing play an important role in the game, because they are strategies for distracting the team trying to guess which opposing players are holding the game pieces (Skeetchestn Indian Band n.d.). The Elder explained how, when drums were taken away as part of cultural suppression, older people came to use sticks in the game instead: "You know, people say [tapping on table], 'Oh it's – that's the way the old people used to do it – bang on the stick when we're playin' that lahal.' The reason they're playing on that, on that stick, is because they took away their drums" (FG 2, 348–49).

The Elders also spoke about loneliness. One woman, who had trained as a licensed practical nurse (LPN), said, "I *had* to leave the reserve, and to leave the reserve I became an LPN, and it was *extremely* lonely" (FG 2,

392–93). One discussed surviving in the "white man's world" in terms of perseverance – "it was tough and you had to get up, dust yourself off, and get on with it" (FG 2, 542–43). Another talked about those who needed to find healing in their own world:

> A lot of the people that I worked with – like, sobered up – were from jails or from the skid rows and stuff like that. They came home and joined our spiritual society, and what they said was "All I ever wanted to do all my life was to come home." (FG 1, 994–97)

For this speaker, the sense of coming home "doesn't only mean the place, you know. It doesn't only mean the place. To come home is to know your belief and feel free again" (FG 1, 1003–4).

Finally, the participants mentioned the importance of helping others to learn more about First Nations people. For example, one Elder spoke about the staff in a residential care facility who decided that her mother had "gone bonkers" (FG 1, 106) when she reverted to Carrier, her own language, presumably because no one on staff could speak it or perhaps even recognize it as a language. The Elder suggested to the staff that the facility should hire a staffer who spoke Carrier. Another Elder explained that "we gotta get the non-Native to not just do the 'poor Indian thing' – they gotta walk with us for about a half a mile or so and learn why people don't wanna see those memories" (FG 2, 476–77). And finally, another talked about the role of the focus group itself in teaching others about First Nations people. He commented that he was glad that

> you [the research team] came and that you listened. Because you understand us, the Native people, a little better than you did before you came. And now it'd be an honour if you could say, "Yes! You know them people are not all that bad, [laughing] not all that stupid after all – especially them old ones!" (FG 2, 2227–35)

Residential Schools: "We Keep Coming Back Here"
Residential schools were often mentioned: as one Elder commented, "we keep coming back here" (FG 1, 976). Thus, the subject warrants separate attention, both because of its relevance for the development of CIRCA-BC and because of the pervasiveness of its ongoing consequences. This was highlighted by one Elder who had attended residential school and who

described his own experiences of "going to courts and going to therapists, and going to ceremonies nearly all my life, trying to fix some of these things up" (FG 1, 763–65). He dismissed the idea "that the past is past, it's all history now" with the reminder that "history isn't over, it's still going" (FG 1, 765, 767).

Although residential school was clearly part of the Elders' shared history, a predominant theme that emerged in their discussion of residential school was the diversity of their experiences in growing up. Only two of the four Elders had attended residential school, while another had not attended any school at all during childhood. The fourth, who was of mixed heritage, attended a school in the town; this emerged when, in response to another participant's comment that she "could pass for a white lady" (FG 1, 479), she said that she "would never pass for a white. They knew who you were ... We got chased home from school every day of the week. Rocks thrown at us, calling us [half]breeds" (FG 1, 480–83).

Elders also mentioned that some individuals – or perhaps groups – were targeted at the residential schools: "these are the people that tried to hang on tightly to the customs and the ways of the language, and the government targeted them and beat them every single day" (FG 1, 492–93). By contrast, "some kids ... were favourites. Pets. So-and-so, because he was so cute, never got touched" (FG 1, 779–81). Elders also discussed differing ways of coping with the school experience: some people were unwilling – or unable – to talk about it, whereas others did. For instance, one Elder compared the reaction of her parents: "Mom *never* wanted to talk about residential school, ever – she just refused" (FG 1, 323–24). When, in her nineties, she finally spoke of it, "the stuff she brought up was horrendous, and the thing is that she never dealt with it ... She would get absolutely hysterical to the point of fainting" (FG 1, 330–33). By contrast, "Dad would tell us stories about what he endured as a child going to school, and he only had three years of it, so he was able to talk about it" (FG 1, 339–41).

Such differences had significant implications for people's ability to cope as survivors. The Elders all agreed on the importance of healing for residential school survivors. In both sessions, they referred to their own healing, including participating in drug and alcohol counselling and healing circles. They also said that the process of healing could be long and difficult, and added that not everyone would, or could, undertake it. One, who knew about the healing activities that the other Elders had done, said to them, "You all worked really hard to get to this level. There's lots of our people who have never sat down and talked about these traumas that happened. They just haven't" (FG 2, 519–21). Another pointed out that "a lot of people can't – can't handle a healing circle" (FG 1, 389). Finally, the Elders acknowledged the implications of the diverse experiences of residential school: "some of those things have to come up one way or another, and it's – we've got to find the language where it doesn't hurt ... where it heals instead of brings up animosity" (FG 1, 769–71).

How Old People Remember: "The Colour of the Rainbow in the Bubble of Water"

In counterpoint to their discussion of memory loss as choosing not to remember, the Elders talked about the importance and value of the process of reminiscing. The woman who had worked as an LPN talked about the orientation that she gave to nurses and caregivers regarding reminiscence with older First Nation people. She highlighted the importance of oral history and collective memory, referring to her mother's reminiscing: "there was nothing wrong with her memory of ancient times, you know, and what they learned at that time, also, she would have been twelve, fifteen then. So the stuff she learned from her grandmother and great-grandparents – the ancient knowledge – they remember" (FG 1, 127–30). She also mentioned the way that old people remember: "old people remember a lot – in infinite detail – of stuff that happened that time, you know, even the colour of the rainbow in the bubble of water, or they'll describe it in a hundred words what that looked like" (FG 1, 120–22). Participants themselves, after having talked about recovering memories through the process of healing from residential school trauma, sometimes evoked their own memories in vivid detail. One Elder recalled a camping trip with his father, weaving details of physical place ("laying in the back of a tent, you know, a regular old, old, old red tent"), of sound ("I can remember hearing my father and the other men out there *laughing,* and it seemed like it was far, far away, but they were just in front of the tent, in front of the fire"), of time ("about six o'clock in the morning, when the sun was coming up"), and of feeling ("you felt really secure") (FG 1, 906–7, 910–12, 912–13, 914). He remembered such moments as "wonderful times that were very innocent before those times of alcoholism and stuff like that. Those are the kind of memories that I want" (FG 1, 921–22).

Elders also talked about the kinds of images that might prompt reminiscing in First Nations seniors. These included subjects from nature, "a trail, or something like that – animals, bears and cougars and fish" (FG 1, 1077), "local mountain and river sites" (FG 2, 917), or images that could appeal to other senses: "Indian rhubarb, pictures of that, you say, 'God, you know, I can *taste* that!' You know, how crunchy nice it is" (FG 1, 1080–81). They also discussed the potential of media such as a television show that depicted life on the West Coast in the 1950s, with one recalling that "Mom and Dad and a whole bunch of people from the reserve used to just *love* to get together and watch it, and then they'd *laugh*. To me, that brought out a history in them because they recognized something" (FG 1, 685–87). Music, too, was suggested, in some cases associated specifically with First Nations people – "some stick game songs even, the old ones, not the new ones" (FG 1, 1088). Other forms of music were also recommended: "I remember some *beautiful* songs that came out just right after the war and during the war ... Some of the songs that they remember – Elvis Presley, Hank Williams" (FG 1, 1097–99). The war itself emerged as a topic for reminiscence: "a lot of people about that age grew up through the war, or the war period. They can tell you the stories" (FG 1, 1131–32).

Elders also drew on their own memories to suggest images, often leading to more reminiscing as others contributed memories evoked by the images. In some cases, this process highlighted that an image could arouse both positive and negative memories for individuals. For example, one Elder talked about First Nations girls doing Highland dancing and recalled that "they were really good" (FG 1, 653). Another commented that though some people might think it was great, "if you brought one of those pictures up, then it covers a lot of things – [like] how good of a job the government was doing on us" (FG 1, 847–48).

Indigenizing CIRCA-BC: "We Have to Be Very Careful"
When considering the needs of First Nations people who might use the CIRCA-BC program, Elders identified two particularly problematic aspects of its format. The first was the feature of random access of generic photos, music, and video clips that are intended for a broad audience rather than for a particular individual. After learning about this feature in the first session, one Elder commented that, because shared reminiscence can be so difficult for residential school survivors, "we have to be very careful how we bring some stuff up" (FG 1, 294). This point was repeatedly made throughout the first session, as Elders expressed the need to "be very selective as to what you can show pictures of" (FG 1, 593–94). One suggested talking with

people before using the program with them and then preselecting pictures: "If you get a group of people with dementia, kind of just, kind of feel things around a bit and say 'okay, he doesn't want to talk about ...'" (FG 1, 599–601). Another recommended that levels be incorporated into the program:

> In terms of presenting materials to different types of personalities that you're dealing with, I think that you need to develop levels, like ten different levels, so that a person with my particular background, who has dealt with all the issues around residential school and oppression can handle pictures in that situation and not go bonkers. But, at the same time, I don't want to be denied those pictures, because they're a part of *my* memory. (FG 1, 666–71)

In general, Elders agreed that, no matter what strategy was used to select materials for particular individuals, giving users the capability to do so was an important feature to include.

The second problematic feature was the division of images into categories. This emerged when Elders were asked which of seven proposed categories would be most appropriate for certain images, such as a picture of traditional net fishing for salmon. One Elder suggested the category of "People, Places, and Events" for that photo, because it was associated with the annual return of the salmon to spawning rivers. However, she then challenged the need for categories at all: "You get too technical. I just want *all* these pictures in here somewhere where I can just click it ... and it'll be there" (FG 2, 1587–91). In her view, categories and the captions that accompanied the photos were labels that were too controlling and could interfere with storytelling, "because we're making up stories when we're talking with the person. 'Do you remember anything like this?' It's a stimulation" (FG 2, 1597–1600).

With reference to the program content, several criteria were cited as important in selecting media. One criterion concerned perspective in the portrayal of First Nations people. Speaking generally about choosing media, one Elder laughed and advised us "not to use the cowboys and Indians kind of thing because they're all white people. They're not our people" (FG 2, 1208–10). She emphasized, "It's not real. What you're trying to show is the reality that used to be part of *my* reality" (FG 2, 1219–21).

A second criterion was familiarity, which was interlaced with themes that arose earlier, including a sense of identity as First Nations people. In some cases, the participants highlighted similarities. For example, in response to a photo of a woman from the Quw'utsun' (Cowichan) Nation holding a traditional Quw'utsun' sweater, one remarked, "it's amazing how the people looked alike, hey? She looks like my mother" (FG 1, 1319–21).[4] Another added, laughing, "she looks like my grandma" (FG 1, 1323). On the other hand, a photo could prompt comments regarding differences: "down Cowichan area, that would be a wonderful picture ... Up here, we don't see those costumes" (FG 1, 1475–77).

Links between identity and place emerged again as a theme. The Elders closely scrutinized some pictures to determine where they might have been taken, extensively discussing their similarities and differences with respect to their own experience. While examining one of these photos, an Elder said, "there's a lot of things that are familiar. One of them is the dress of our people ... the old saddles there, the horse ... But the kids got short hair" (FG 1, 1573–80). This led to an exchange about who might most appreciate the shot: "for the Coast this'd be okay," with another adding, "or even the Prairies" (FG 1, 1581–82). However, despite these acknowledgments of differences, the Elders generally recommended keeping such pictures for the CIRCA-BC program. One stated, "My mom likes to see other culture and, you know, especially Native. It's beautiful that our people still do these things" (FG 1, 1483–84).

In summary, Elders raised several issues and cautions to consider in adapting CIRCA-BC for First Nations people. At the same time, they cited the importance of finding ways to support positive reminiscing for First Nations people with dementia, because, as one participant noted, it could bring them "half an hour of happiness, of thinking and remembering" (FG 2, 1151).

Reflections on What We Learned

We began our study seeking guidance from First Nations Elders, first, about how best to represent First Nations people in a CIRCA-BC program and, second, about using the program with First Nations people with dementia. What we learned gave us insight into these two topics, but it also led us to a topic beyond these, inviting us to think about how our underlying assumptions about CIRCA-BC could be reframed in light of Elders' perspectives.

With respect to representation, Walsh (2008) has drawn attention to the perspectives of colonization that are prevalent in publicly archived media representations of First Nations people from the early part of the twentieth century. Like Walsh, the Elders in our study both recognized and contested this colonization perspective. Their comments regarding "cowboys and Indians," and the idea that an image could show "how good of a job the government was doing on us," resonate with other First Nation views about the use of media as a tool for colonization, particularly in residential schools (see, for example, "Akipoulala" in Gaudet and Louttit 2014, 91–92). This, coupled with the Elders' interest in helping non–First Nations people to understand more about First Nation people, highlights the importance of seeking their guidance to ensure that the CIRCA-BC program would not perpetuate colonizing perspectives.

Fortunately, not all the photos that we located were grounded in colonizing ideology. The Elders' discussion of several shots, particularly those showing First Nations people engaged in traditional activities, suggested that they were consistent with First Nations views. At the same time, the question of *which* nation was depicted was obviously important, as revealed in Elders' debates about which people might most appreciate certain photos. Margaret Kovach's (2009, 37) discussion of Indigenous epistemologies is relevant here. She claims that Indigenous knowledges are contextualized to tribal affiliations because they are tied to place but that Indigenous people generally understand each other because they share common beliefs about the world. Our findings agreed with this statement. In general, the Elders recommended that we retain most of the photos that were not taken in their own territory. They felt that doing so would make the program more relevant for First Nations people from other regions but also that, even where local traditions differed, there was often sufficient overlap to prompt a broad sense of familiarity. Nevertheless, the importance of place suggests that it would be useful to seek guidance from Elders who are most familiar with the territory of the people for whom the program is intended.

Determining which media to include was also relevant to our question about whether CIRCA-BC would be suitable for First Nations people with dementia. In our broader study, we were exploring ways to develop a program that could be used widely for all long-time residents of British Columbia, including First Nations people and people from various settler communities. For that reason, we were interested in Elders views' about the relevance of media that were not specific to First Nations and that had been selected by participants from the earlier focus groups in the same region (see Purves et al. 2015). Elders' suggestions for additional media and their comments regarding media selected by the earlier groups revealed considerable overlap in opinions across the groups about what was familiar and appropriate for the program. This is perhaps not surprising, in view of their overlapping histories in time and place.

However, the question of whether CIRCA-BC was suitable for First Nations people with dementia entailed more than identifying appropriate media. Here, the Elders' broad, intertwined understandings of individual memory loss emerged as more relevant than the single strand of dementia, which they generally saw as a European disease, relatively uncommon in their communities (see also Hulko et al. 2010). It is not surprising, then, that their discussion of using CIRCA-BC for people with memory loss reflected common understandings in their communities – the traditional view of memory loss as part of aging and the more recent view of memory loss as suppression of traumas associated with residential school.

Nor is it surprising that these understandings were associated with mixed views about CIRCA-BC. The Elders acknowledged the positive aspects of reminiscing with old people, but, and perhaps more urgently, they emphasized the risks for those who could not cope with traumatic memories. Their suggestions concerning the need to use CIRCA-BC carefully, including tailoring it to accommodate differing experiences, may be challenging to implement fully, given the design of the program. Nonetheless, their recommendations about getting to know a person before using the program and about preselecting media (perhaps, for example, by omitting the thematic category titled "School Days") offer a starting point.

The themes that arose during the focus group sessions also invited us to consider the ways in which we could reframe our underlying assumptions about CIRCA-BC. Specifically, the Elders' comments about collective memory preservation and loss, storytelling, place, and the importance of intergenerational sharing of knowledge drove us to re-evaluate our preexisting focus on reminiscence as a strategy to support social conversations for people with dementia. In doing so, we recognize the centrality of storytelling as a traditional way of sharing collective memory across generations. Thus, keeping in mind Elders' comments about old people remembering ancient knowledge, we propose that storytelling could be a starting point in using CIRCA-BC with First Nations people. For example, the program could be assessed for its ability to elicit stories and to promote storytelling intergenerationally. The emergence of place as a key theme is also important, consistent with Kovach's (2009) claim that, in contrast to the temporal orientation of Western narrative, place is the primary orientation in

Indigenous storytelling. This again highlights the necessity of considering the representation of place from the perspectives of the First Nations people who might use the program and, in evaluating its use with them, of attending carefully to their responses to place.

In conclusion, our findings, constrained though they are by the fact that our sample size was small and that all four participants lived in the same region, offer valuable guidance in our ongoing development of CIRCA-BC. At present, whether the program can benefit older First Nations adults with memory loss remains a question for future research. Nevertheless, our study has provided us with rich insights into how that question should be explored and perhaps even reframed: Can we create a program that will give older First Nations adults with memory loss a feeling, if only for half an hour, of coming home?

Notes

1   We use "Elder" for our research participants, and we refer to all older adults who are Indigenous as "older First Nation (or Indigenous) adults." This is for clarity's sake rather than to denote that our participants are traditional knowledge keepers and others are not. "Elder" is the preferred language for all older First Nation adults (see Introduction, this volume).

2   To protect the privacy of the four people who participated in this study, we have chosen not to attribute quotes to specific individuals. Instead, we cite focus group sessions (FG 1 or FG 2) and line numbers to ensure authenticity.

3   "Lights went out" is a phrase from the study by Wendy Hulko et al. (2010). Although the Elder quoted in this chapter participated in that study as well, it was introduced there by a different Elder.

4   The Quw'utsun' Nation is situated in the Cowichan Valley on Vancouver Island, some distance west from the area of our study.

References

Alm, Norman, Arlene Astell, Maggie Ellis, Richard Dye, Gary Gowans, and Jim Campbell. 2004. "A Cognitive Prosthesis and Communication Support for People with Dementia." *Neuropsychological Rehabilitation* 14 (1–2): 117–34.

Astell, Arlene J., Maggie P. Ellis, Lauren Bernardi, Norman Alm, Richard Dye, Gary Gowans, and Jim Campbell. 2010. "Using a Touch Screen Computer to Support Relationships between People with Dementia and Caregivers." *Interactive Computing* 22 (4): 267–75.

Fels, Deborah I., and Arlene J. Astell. 2011. "Storytelling as a Model of Conversation for People with Dementia and Caregivers." *American Journal of Alzheimer's Disease and Other Dementias* 26 (7): 535–41.

Fromholt, P., and S.F. Larsen. 1992. "Autobiographical Memory and Life-History

Narratives in Aging and Dementia (Alzheimer's Type)." In *Theoretical Perspectives on Autobiographical Memory,* ed. M. Conway, D. Rubin, H. Spinnler, and W. Wagenaar, 413–26. Dordrecht, NL: Kluwer Academic.

Garvey, Gail, Donna Simmonds, Vanessa Clements, Peter O'Rourke, Karen Sullivan, Don Gorman, Venessa Curnow, Susi Wise, and Elizabeth Beattie. 2011. "Making Sense of Dementia: Understanding amongst Indigenous Australians." *International Journal of Geriatric Psychiatry* 26 (6): 649–56.

Gaudet, Janice Cindy, and William Louttit. 2014. "Is There Hope?" In *Reconciliation and the Way Forward: Collected Essays and Personal Reflections,* ed. Shelagh Rogers, Mike DeGagné, Glen Lowry, and Sara Fryer, 85–100. Ottawa: Aboriginal Healing Foundation.

Henderson, J. Neil. 2002. "The Experience and Interpretation of Dementia: Cross-Cultural Perspectives." *Journal of Cross-Cultural Gerontology* 17 (3): 195–96.

Henderson, J. Neil, and L. Carson Henderson. 2002. "Cultural Construction of Disease: A 'Supernormal' Construct of Dementia in an American Indian Tribe." *Journal of Cross-Cultural Gerontology* 17 (3): 197–212.

Hendrix, Levanne R., and Fr. Hank Swift Cloud-Lebeau. 2006. "Working with American Indian Families: Collaboration with Families for the Care of Older American Indians with Memory Loss." In *Ethnicity and the Dementias,* 2nd ed., ed. Gwen Yeo and Dolores Gallagher-Thompson, 147–62. New York: Routledge.

Hulko, Wendy, Evelyn Camille, Elisabeth Antifeau, Mike Arnouse, Nicole Bachynksi, and Denise Taylor. 2010. "Views of First Nation Elders on Memory Loss and Memory Care in Later Life." *Journal of Cross-Cultural Gerontology* 25 (4): 317–42. DOI:10.1007/s10823-010-9123-9.

Hulko, Wendy, and Louise Stern. 2009. "Cultural Safety, Decision-Making and Dementia: Troubling Notions of Autonomy and Personhood." In *Decision-Making, Personhood and Dementia: Exploring the Interface,* ed. Deborah O'Connor and Barbara Purves, 70–87. London: Jessica Kingsley.

Jacklin, K., W. Warry, and J. Pace. 2012. "Using Participatory Approaches to Explore Aboriginal Understandings of Dementia and Dementia Care." *Gerontologist* 52 (suppl. 1): 458.

Kim, Esther S., Stuart J. Cleary, Tammy Hopper, Kathryn Bayles, Nidhi Mahendra, Tamiko Azuma, and Audette Rackley. 2006. "Evidence-Based Practice Recommendations for Working with Individuals with Dementia: Group Reminiscence Therapy." *Journal of Medical Speech-Language Pathology* 14 (3): 23–35.

Kovach, Margaret. 2009. *Indigenous Methodologies: Characteristics, Conversations, and Contexts.* Toronto: University of Toronto Press.

Lanting, Shawnda, Margaret Crossley, Debra Morgan, and Allison Cammer. 2011. "Aboriginal Experiences of Aging and Dementia in a Context of Sociocultural Change: Qualitative Analysis of Key Informant Group Interviews with Aboriginal Seniors." *Journal of Cross-Cultural Gerontology* 26 (1): 103–17.

Luborsky, Mark R. 1994. "The Identification and Analysis of Themes and Patterns." In *Qualitative Methods in Aging Research,* ed. Jaber F. Gubrium and Andrea Sankar, 189–210. Thousand Oaks, CA: Sage.

O'Connor, Deborah, Alison Phinney, and Wendy Hulko. 2010. "Dementia at the Intersections: A Unique Case Study Exploring Social Location." *Journal of Aging Studies* 24 (1): 30–39.

Pollitt, P.A. 1997. "The Problem of Dementia in Australian Aboriginal and Torres Strait Islander Communities." *International Journal of Geriatric Psychiatry* 12: 155–63.

Purves, Barbara A., Alison Phinney, Wendy Hulko, Gloria Puurveen, and Arlene J. Astell. 2015. "Developing CIRCA-BC and Exploring the Role of the Computer as a Third Participant in Conversation." *American Journal of Alzheimer's Disease and Other Dementias* 30 (1): 101–7. DOI:10.1177/1533317514539031.

Skeetchestn Indian Band. N.d. "Lahal." http://www.skeetchestn.ca/lahal.

Sutherland, M. 2007. *Alzheimer's Disease and Related Dementias within Aboriginal Individuals: Roundtable Forum.* Toronto: Alzheimer Society of Ontario.

TRC (Truth and Reconciliation Commission of Canada). 2015. *Honouring the Truth, Reconciling for the Future: Summary of the Final Report of the Truth and Reconciliation Commission of Canada.* Ottawa: Truth and Reconciliation Commission of Canada. http://nctr.ca/assets/reports/Final%20Reports/Executive_Summary_English_Web.pdf.

Walsh, Andrea. 2008. "Re-placing History: Critiquing the Colonial Gaze through Photographic Works by Jeffrey Thomas and Greg Staats." In *Locating Memory: Photographic Acts*, ed. Annette Kuhn and Kirsten Emiko McAllister, 21–51. New York: Berghahn Books.

CHAPTER 9

FOCUS(ING) ON LOVE AND RESPECT

Translating Elders' Teachings on Aging and Memory Loss into Learning Tools for Children and Youth

Wendy Hulko, Danielle Wilson, and Jessica Kent

ELDERS ARE HIGHLY VALUED in many Indigenous nations as the guardians of traditional knowledge and teachers of younger generations (Archibald 2008; Carter 2012; Crowe-Salazar 2007; Mehl-Madrona 2009), largely through oral means such as storytelling. However, many Canadian First Nations are losing their traditional teachings, in part due to disconnections between youth and Elders (Mack and Hulko 2013) and the diminished role of storytelling. This is the result of contemporary colonizing practices whereby Indigenous children were taken into state care via residential schools and foster homes. Historically, storytelling has been an important form of knowledge exchange among Canadian First Nations (Archibald 2008; Battiste 2013), and grassroots efforts are being made to bring back and/or strengthen it. Many First Nations have also adopted mainstream teaching tools, such as storybooks and videos, which can be a useful means of preserving the knowledge of Elders and honouring traditional teachings.

In the past, Elders educated children and youth, and many still perform this role in their communities. Nowadays, they are still referred to as traditional knowledge keepers and often asked to share their cultural knowledge. However, their participation in addressing contemporary issues such as dementia, HIV/AIDS, environmental stewardship, and community connectedness may be limited if they are viewed solely as keepers of tradition. Elders have an important role to play in bringing forward knowledge of the past and applying or bridging it to contemporary issues, thereby creating new understandings of dementia and other culturally appropriate teachings.

This chapter focuses on a project titled "Stories of Our Past: A Dementia Knowledge Translation Project between First Nations Elders and Children," as an example of how this type of bridging – across generations and time – can lead to new knowledge. From June 2012 to July 2013, the research team collaborated with Elders from the Secwepemc Nation to produce a storybook for children and a video for youth, both of which focused on dementia, to help Secwepemc young people learn about aging and memory loss. As part of the Stories of Our Past knowledge translation and exchange (KTE) project, those who were shown these teaching tools were asked to fill out a questionnaire. The themes derived from its open-ended queries were how successfully the book and video incorporated Secwepemc perspectives, whether they strengthened relationships between youth and Elders, and how well they encouraged learning. In all, the book and the video were well received, offering a solid foundation upon which to build future research and education.

Culturally Specific Educational Materials on Aging and Memory Loss

Aging and memory loss is a new area of teaching for First Nations schools, just as it is a relatively new area of Indigenous research (see Introduction, this volume). Indeed, when Stories of Our Past was launched, culturally specific educational materials regarding the topic did not exist. A number of storybooks about dementia have been written for children between the ages of four and twelve (Alzheimer Society of Canada 2014), most of which present a grandmother living with dementia. Only a few of them reflect the traditions and beliefs of minority ethnic and/or racialized communities: these include *Grandfather's Story Cloth* (Gerdner 2008), *Singing with Momma Lou* (Jacobs Altman and Johnson 2002), *Wordsworth Dances the Waltz* (Kakugawa and DeSica 2007), and *Getting to Know Ruben Plotnick* (Rosenbluth 2005). A bilingual book, *Grandfather's Story Cloth*, was created specifically for Hmong children; *Singing with Momma Lou* features an African American grandmother reflecting on the civil rights era; the main character in *Wordsworth Dances the Waltz* is a Hawaiian mouse; and *Getting to Know Ruben Plotnick* focuses on a Jewish grandmother who has dementia.

These books are not directed at First Nations children, and none include Indigenous characters. To our knowledge, *The Gathering Tree* (Loyie and Brissenden 2012) is the only health-related book created for First Nations children. First published in 2005, it addresses HIV/AIDS in a First Nations family and is intended to be used as a teaching tool by educators and community members. After Stories of Our Past was completed and our storybook was released, a Tahltan Elder wrote *The Mind Thief,* a graphic novel on Alzheimer's disease, through a collaboration with the National Core for Neuroethics (Framst and Harvey 2015).

Jill Manthorpe (2005, 313) argues that "exploration of material written for and about children and dementia offers a wealth of opportunities for what is called 'dementia' and its close association with context." Indeed, the creation of materials about dementia and Secwepemc Elders could shape how Secwepemc children and youth, and possibly other Indigenous people, view and respond to dementia and aging. This creation of dementia knowledge translation tools exemplifies "partnership and multidirectional communication" (Illes, Chahal, and Beattie 2011, 262) and could "begin to cure the cultural context in which we experience dementia" (Basting 2009, 70). These tools can support teaching and learning in Indigenous communities, while also contesting the dominant discourse on dementia, which presents it as pathological and sees those who experience it as incapable, mere shadows of their former selves (see Hulko 2009). According to Anne Basting (2009) and others, this culture needs to be cured. Tools based on the belief systems of Indigenous communities may depict dementia as a normal part of aging and/or as a consequence of colonization. They will also present persons with dementia as worthy of love and respect, like any valued citizen or Elder.

To our knowledge, there are no educational videos regarding dementia that are intended for First Nations youth. Moreover, videos on Indigenous people and dementia are uncommon. Three examples of the latter include *Love in the Time of Dementia,* an animated film narrated in English and Anindilyakwa, the language spoken by the Warnindhilyagwa people of northern Australia, which is directed at family members caring for someone with dementia (Smith n.d.); Neil Henderson's video on American Indian Elders and dementia, also created for care partners and health care professionals (Pace, Boesch, and Jacklin 2010); and *Alzheimer's Disease: Stories from Caregivers,* produced for the Native American Outreach Program of the Banner Alzheimer's Institute (Banner Alzheimer's Institute 2010).

An example of Internet-based media on dementia, which targets non-Indigenous Canadian children and youth, is *When Dementia Is in the House* (Nichols and Chow 2011). It tells the story of a family whose mother is living with frontotemporal degeneration, and it has an accompanying online activity book for children (Chow and Elliot 2012). Both were developed by Dr. Tiffany Chow and her colleagues in Ontario through the support of the Canadian Dementia Knowledge Translation Network, which also funded Stories of Our Past.

Youth of today access information largely through the Internet (Statistics Canada 2013), including via video, which is a common online format. Elders are less likely than youth to use the Internet (Statistics Canada 2013), a difference that potentially contributes to the disconnection between them. Thus, there is an opportunity for Elders to use modern communication methods, such as videos and other resources shared online, to teach First Nations youth about contemporary issues.

Development and Evaluation of the Teaching Tools

After we completed research with the Secwepemc Nation on memory loss and memory care (Hulko et al., 2010), Elders identified a gap in the educational resources of community schools for younger children (John Jules, pers. comm., January 26, 2012). Elders recommended the creation of materials on caring for "grandma and grandpa," which would be grounded in traditional Secwepemc views on aging (Evelyn Camille, pers. comm., January 26, 2012). The research team, including the Elder advisers, saw the development of this material as a tangible gift for the communities that had contributed to the study, consistent with Indigenous customs. Thus, Stories of Our Past is an example of reciprocity, which is a key principle of doing collaborative research with Indigenous communities (Kovach 2010; Varcoe et al. 2011; Wilson 2008).

Stories of Our Past was connected to a community-based research project titled "Culturally Safe Dementia Care: Building Nursing Capacity to Care for First Nation Elders with Memory Loss" (Hulko et al. 2014). Both projects represent an ongoing collaboration between Secwepemc Elders, researchers, and practitioners; for Stories of Our Past, this included First Nation artists (Karlene Harvey and Trevor Mack) and educators. The two artists had family members with dementia and thus had a personal and professional commitment to the project. To orient them to the project and ensure that both the book and the video reflected the study findings, the research team shared an article and two storybooks with them. The article, by Wendy Hulko et al. (2010), discussed earlier research with Secwepemc Elders on memory loss, and the two storybooks were *Singing with Momma Lou* and *Wordsworth Dances the Waltz.* Jessica Kent, who was a bachelor of social work practicum student with Stories of Our Past and a research assistant for the Culturally Safe Dementia Care (CSDC) project, met with the artists frequently and became a co-producer of the video.

The resulting twenty-two-minute video, *Remembering Our Way Forward: Dementia from a Secwepemc Perspective,* and twenty-four-page storybook, *A Good Day with Grandma (Kyé7e) and Me,* were to be shared online and in DVD and book formats. They were developed through the filming of two of the eight roundtable discussions held with Secwepemc communities for the CSDC project, which had a total sample of thirty-four Elders. Ten individual interviews were also conducted for Stories of Our Past. Once Karlene Harvey and Trevor Mack had created draft versions of the storybook and video, a focus group session was held with the Elder advisers and two of this chapter's authors. The drafts were revised to ensure that they reflected findings from earlier collaborative research with Secwepemc Elders (Hulko et al. 2010) and that they emphasized specific Secwepemc cultural traditions, such as sharing food. For example, the image in Figure 9.1, which depicts the family eating breakfast, was added following this focus group.

The revised versions were then shared with teachers and school officials. All seventeen Secwepemc communities and ten of their schools were invited to view them and give feedback through anonymous questionnaires and consultation sessions. Only three of the seventeen expressed interest in providing feedback, all of which had participated in the CSDC project. At two Secwepemc schools in the south (near Kamloops) and one in the north (near Williams Lake), the teachers completed the questionnaire.[1] Next, three consultation sessions were held with Elders and other community members, who also filled out the questionnaire. Two pages in length, it included four Likert-like scales (from 1 [strongly disagree] to 5 [strongly agree]) and seven open-ended questions (see Table 9.1). Analysis of these quantitative and qualitative data allowed us to evaluate the project, particularly to determine how well the storybook and the video reflected Secwepemc perspectives on aging and memory loss and strengthened intergenerational relationships,

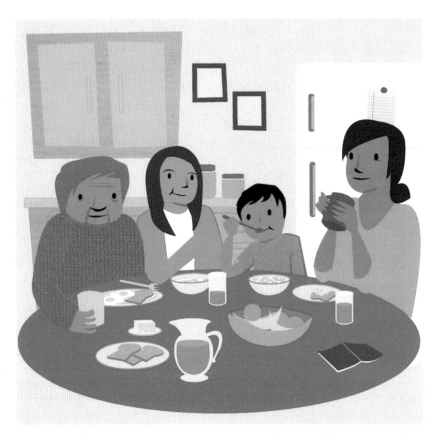

FIGURE 9.1 In this scene from *A Good Day with Grandma (Kyé7e) and Me*, the grandmother (left) sits with her two grandchildren, Lisa and Ben, and their mother.

the first two themes of the study. The third theme, that of learning outcomes, arose from our inductive analysis of the data. This entailed reviewing responses in the qualitative section of the questionnaire and looking for themes among them. Although the questionnaire did not directly ask participants to identify what they had learned or hoped that others would learn from the book and the video, their responses often addressed this subject.

We calculated simple descriptive statistics for the quantitative responses: the average score and the range of scores for each of the four questions. The replies from the two sets of respondents (teachers and community members) regarding the storybook and the video were scrutinized for statements that reflected "intergenerational connectedness and Secwepemc perspectives on aging and memory loss" or "ways to improve the tools."

Feedback on the Teaching Tools

Who Took Part and How They Scored the Tools

The sample for the KTE evaluation was composed of twenty-nine people who worked and/or lived in one of four Secwepemc communities. Fifty-two percent of them (fifteen individuals) were teachers, and 48 percent (fourteen people) were community members. Eighty-six percent of the twenty-nine participants were First Nations (only two teachers and two community members were not).

Our evaluation showed that participants strongly supported the two teaching tools, as detailed in Table 9.1. On a five-point scale, The average scores by teachers on the utility and novelty of the storybook and video ranged from 3.40 (utility – storybook) and 3.25 (novelty – storybook) to 3.65 (utility and novelty – video) to 4.83 (utility and novelty – teaching tool not specified). The fact that the scores were higher when the tool was not specified, for both the teachers and the community members, is interesting and could be due to the value placed on education by Indigenous communities in Canada (see Battiste 2013). None of the fourteen community members specified which tool (video or storybook) they were rating, and their average scores ranged from 4.57 (practicality and utility) to 4.79 (novelty). In Table 9.1, the figures in parentheses indicate the range of responses, from 1 (strongly disagree) to 5 (strongly agree). Only five of the table's sixteen cells show a score of lower than 3, and three of these are for utility. The range of average scores for the practicality of the book and the video was 3.75 to 4.67, and it was 3.17 to 4.80 for their applicability. The written comments, all of which were positive, indicated that the tools contributed to the exchange of intergenerational knowledge, as will be seen below.

Expressed Support for the Teaching Tools

In addition to these high average scores on the four Likert-type scales, written and oral statements collected from the surveys and consultations also expressed strong support for the teaching tools. As mentioned, we asked seven open-ended questions, three of which were the following:

- Please comment on the clarity and respectfulness with which the issues raised in the book/film were treated.

- Did you feel that this book/film could be used as an educational tool for children to better understand aging and memory loss of their grandparents and other Elders?
- What could have been improved upon within this book/film?

Remarks made during the feedback sessions relate to the three themes – incorporating Secwepemc perspectives on aging and memory loss, strengthening intergenerational relationships, and generating learning outcomes – as detailed below. The first two themes were stated goals of the Stories of Our Past project and were therefore explicitly assessed. As we analyzed the completed questionnaires, we noticed that learning outcomes were frequently mentioned, so this became a third theme.

TABLE 9.1 Ratings of teaching tools

	Teachers (n = 15)			Community members (n = 14)
	Storybook	Video	Both tools (non-specific)	Both tools (non-specific)
Utility (useful education tool for children)	3.40 (1–5)	3.67 (2–5)	4.83 (4–5)	4.57 (2–5)
Novelty (introduces new material from a Secwepemc perspective)	3.25 (1–5)	3.67 (3–5)	4.83 (4–5)	4.79 (3–5)
Practicality (shows practical way for children and youth to help)	3.75 (3–5)	4.00 (3–5)	4.67 (4–5)	4.57 (3–5)
Applicability (plan to use in my future teaching practice)	3.50 (3–5)	3.17 (1–5)	4.80 (4–5)	4.67 (3–5)

NOTE: 1 = strongly disagree, 5 = strongly agree

Secwepemc Perspectives on Aging and Memory Loss

With respect to the introduction of Secwepemc perspectives on aging and memory loss, many responses reinforced what we had learned about Secwepemc values during the roundtable discussions with Elders. These teaching points include, for example, the importance of maintaining connections between families, communities, and Elders; developing relationships based on love, trust, and respect; and keeping people active and involved in their own care. For instance, the importance of maintaining family ties appears in the storybook when Kyé7e moves into her daughter's house after leaving her home on the reserve. Kyé7e's granddaughter Lisa tells her younger brother Ben that "Kyé7e needs to be close to her family now" (Harvey and Hulko 2013, 2).

Throughout our research with Secwepemc communities, preserving links with family and community was stressed repeatedly as a priority. An elementary teacher at Adams Lake Indian Reserve 4 expressed their agreement with the project's promotion of this value: "As a community, we need to reconnect with family/extended family. People need to feel a part of a family/community." Maintaining ties with Elders is challenging in many Secwepemc communities because Elders who require comprehensive care must often move to a larger centre, as a Soda Creek Elder pointed out: "Yes, young people have to understand, most people live in homes not at their personal home community." To our knowledge, despite much interest, none of the seventeen Secwepemc communities has developed its own residential care facility.

Retaining a connection to family and community is also understood in cultural terms. The importance of keeping Elders and youth connected to their culture was discussed in the video. Elder Barb Larson emphasized that traditions are part of *"our survival"* (Mack and Hulko 2013). Also in the film, Elder Evelyn Camille shows viewers her sweat lodge and describes the ceremony that takes place within (Mack and Hulko 2013). Feedback from respondents affirmed that the teaching tools were effective in relaying cultural ideals and values. A commentator from Rosie Seymour Elementary said, "[the storybook] covers all the bases: family, children, animals." A non–First Nations teacher at Sorrento remarked that the "explanation [of the] full circle [of life] is great [in the video]."[2] And an educator at Switsemalph Indian Reserve 6 in Salmon Arm suggested that "[these tools will help] to keep our knowledge and culture alive."

In line with Secwepemc values, the type of care that Elders receive should be based on love, trust, and respect. For example, the storybook highlights the importance of patience as family members help Kyé7e feel safe and calm (Harvey and Hulko 2013). Many respondents recognized these values in the teaching tools and affirmed their agreement. A community health nurse in Williams Lake who is a member of the Nlaka'pamux Nation stated, "[These tools] showed the respect that the people still give the Elders even though they may not remember." A non–First Nations bus driver in Williams Lake said, "I liked the focus on love and respect."

Keeping Elders active and involved relates to family and community connections, and to ways care can be delivered. In the video, Elder Anne Michel encourages youth to keep Elders active by engaging with them. She suggests that they go to their Elders and assures them that they will not bother them. As she explains, Elders "want to be noticed and needed" (Mack and Hulko 2013). The video stresses the importance of culturally meaningful ways through which people can keep their brains active and healthy, including participating in traditional ceremony, which requires memory work, and telling stories (Mack and Hulko 2013). Participants also emphasized the importance of keeping active and healthy. A Nlaka'pamux educator who was born in Chase stated, "Keeping healthy – emotionally, mentally, spiritually, physically – good. Responsibility to maintain own health – good." And an elementary teacher at Adams Lake Indian Reserve 4 said, "Yes, [this is] an important topic, NOT just physical health/nutrition, etc."

Strengthening Intergenerational Relationships

Another central goal of Stories of Our Past was to create tools that could assist in strengthening intergenerational relationships. In the storybook, the grandmother lives with her extended family, and the plot provides examples of how young people can spend time with their older relatives (Harvey and Hulko 2013). In the video, Elders speak to youth about memory loss and aging and how to form healthy relationships with older people (Mack and Hulko 2013). Thus, the video enabled them to speak directly to youth about what aging was like and how to treat Elders with love and respect.

Several teachers, one principal, and one community member commented on how well the tools contributed to intergenerational knowledge exchange through their references to the younger generation, including both their children and grandchildren. Their remarks confirmed a goal of the project in that strengthening intergenerational relationships was a priority for some community members. For example, a Xat'sull culture teacher said, "The younger generation will know [what] to expect and understand what to do about [an Elder becoming forgetful]." A Sugar Cane Elder who is a cultural teacher stated, "[The teaching tools] will help my grandkids to understand dementia better." And a Shuswap Elder who is a caregiver and lives in the community noted that "my children and grandchildren will understand me more."

Respondents also reiterated the importance of strengthening intergenerational relationships, which confirmed their endorsement of this goal. The non–First Nations principal of Rosie Seymour Elementary in Canoe Creek said, it's "important to connect despite illness and that younger people are able to accept and embrace Elders." In Williams Lake, a Tsilhqot'in Aboriginal patient navigator said, "Youth definitely need to understand dementia and [how] it affects the family/Elder." An elementary teacher at Adams Lake Indian Reserve 4 pointed out that the storybook could be used as an activity that Elders and youth do together "if sléle/kyé7e [grandfather or grandmother] reads [to the students] at storytime."

Learning Outcomes

Participants also used the qualitative section to identify learning outcomes in terms of what they took away from the teaching tools and what they felt youth needed to know. They mentioned helping youth understand dementia and how to care for Elders, as well as the importance of certain qualities, such as patience and respect. For example, the storybook emphasizes understanding when Ben's mom and sister Lisa explain to him what it might be like for Kyé7e to forget things and how frustrating that would be (Harvey and Hulko 2013). A Sugar Cane Elder who is a cultural teacher said, "a person looks normal, but [can] forget they asked a question and ask again and again, so patience must be taught to [the] young." A Canoe Creek, Alkali (Esketemc) Elder who works at the school said, "[This project] was good and [the tools] could relate to what happen[s] to people with dementia." This same participant remarked on the personal effectiveness of these teaching tools, indicating that they conveyed information on dementia in a culturally relevant way: "[these teaching tools] helped me understand [dementia] more, so I have more understanding and [will] not get so scared of it."

Other respondents focused on what they saw as important for youth to learn from the video and storybook. A Chase language teacher who lives in Salmon Arm said, "Youth have to understand memory loss of their kyé7es and slé7es and not make fun of them." Another teacher in Chase who is Neskonlith and Nuu-chah-nulth indicated that "respect for our people/ Elders in any case – learning to show respect" was the key learning to be taken from the storybook and video.

We asked respondents, "Why do you feel that knowledge exchange between generations is important to your community and how did this film/storybook contribute to knowledge exchange?" A Nlaka'pamux educator who was born in Chase quoted Elder Ralph Phillips, who appeared in the film: "You do know your culture – how you raise your kids is culture." This remark suggests that knowledge exchange is important because it will influence how the next generation raises its own children, thereby retaining culture.

Although we have separated the three themes to discuss specific aspects of our evaluation, it should be apparent that they often overlap. For example, strengthening intergenerational relationships is inseparable from maintaining a connection to family and community, as well as keeping Elders active. Further, the goals of strengthening relationships and reinforcing cultural perspectives are reflected in the learning outcomes, which include treating Elders with respect.

Release and Uptake of the Teaching Tools

The final versions of the storybook and the film were released in July 2013 at a public forum that was part of a roundtable forum on Indigenous people and dementia, which was co-hosted by two of the authors. Beforehand, however, we incorporated the valuable participant feedback into the two teaching tools: thus, we adjusted the storybook's target audience from kindergarten to Grade 4 to Grades 3 to 6, we contributed funds from the CSDC project to budget for the expected increased demand for copies of the tools, and we changed the community names on the storybook map from colloquial to traditional ones. Fortunately, we managed to fund three production cycles of the storybook and film, as both have generated a great deal of interest from various groups and individuals. This too indicates their usefulness and applicability. Although they were created specifically for Secwepemc schools, other stakeholder groups, including community members, health care staff, and non-First Nations persons, have displayed an interest in them. For example, a colleague of the first author, who had a relative with dementia, expressed his appreciation for the messages in the book and noted the applicability beyond First Nations communities (Chris Walmsley, pers. comm., July 4, 2013). Further, at the public forum in July 2013 and other community events where we distributed the storybook, attendees inquired about purchasing additional copies. As a result, both the film and the book were made freely downloadable through the Thompson Rivers University website, and the book was also available through Research

Gate. As of May 28, 2018, the video had been viewed 325 times on YouTube, and the storybook was accessed through the Thompson Rivers website 7,869 times between November 28, 2013, and September 5, 2014.[3]

The demand for these teaching tools, together with the positive results of the evaluation, indicates that the incorporation of traditional teachings into mediums such as storybooks and videos is an acceptable and supported means of knowledge translation in Secwepemc communities. Moreover, the book and video served as a bridge between Elders and younger people; the knowledge of the former was honoured and translated to learning tools via mediums with which youth are familiar. Thus, in working collaboratively with First Nations, this research demonstrates that knowledge translation projects can support traditional values and beliefs while serving as learning tools for youth and spanning the cultural divide between generations.

These knowledge translation tools served their intended purpose: to raise awareness and understanding of dementia. With increasing rates of dementia among First Nations in Canada (see Introduction, this volume), such teaching tools are necessary to prepare young persons to provide comprehensive care for Elders. The latter are the knowledge keepers of their communities, and a circle of care between Elders and younger people is important to support continued cultural strength and family cohesion.

Limitations

Although all the Secwepemc community schools were invited to participate in the study, only three did so, which limited the representativeness of our sample. Further, we did not seek feedback on the final products and did not track their distribution after we mailed copies to all of the schools and distributed them at public events. The assumption underpinning this project, that children and youth did not have an understanding of aging and memory loss from a Secwepemc perspective, was based on advice from Elders. We did not measure or assess this claim in any way. Lastly, some of the changes suggested at the community consultation sessions, particularly those from teachers, could not be acted upon. This was mainly due to funding limitations and the late point at which we received the feedback. For example, the suggestion was made that youth should participate in the film so that it would include their views and that it should also show an example in which they assisted Elders. Additional – and unanticipated – content was also requested, such as more concrete information on dementia or "coping" with someone who has memory loss, an explanation of medical terms, and the phonetic pronunciation of the Secwepemctsín words such as Kyé7e.

Conclusion and Implications for Research and Education

Although the storybook features a grandmother and grandchildren, much like other children's books on dementia, and there are various videos that examine dementia in an Indigenous context, the two teaching tools are nonetheless unique. Moreover, they avoid pan-indigenizing, as evidenced by participant endorsement of their portrayal of Secwepemc culture and traditions. This nation-specific focus includes the adoption of a holistic approach and the use of the Secwepemcstín language. Further, the demand for copies exceeded our expectations, and the results of the evaluation supported the twin goals of the project. Thus, Stories of Our Past demonstrated that it is possible to change views about and responses to dementia and those living with memory loss, diminished judgment, and behavioural changes in later life. Further, it is possible to expand the public discourse on dementia through artistic creations (see Basting 2009).

In terms of implications for education, this project was originally intended as a gift from researchers and Elders to the community schools, and we recommend that future teaching tool development involve teachers and students from the beginning to incorporate their views and perspectives more thoroughly. This will ensure that the tools have a meaningful impact and durable legacy for future generations and that they will align with the curriculum and other educational initiatives. Further, researchers should consider the creation of knowledge translation tools early on, such as when drafting their grant proposals, and funders like the Canadian Institutes of Health Research should provide resources for KTE tools that are requested or envisioned by communities. In other words, teaching and learning tools that meet community needs can be a manifestation of reciprocity, as in this project.

As to the inclusion of medical information about dementia in children's books, this appears at the end of *Grandma* (Shepherd 2014), a book about a white majority ethnic family, but it is not included in *A Good Day with Grandma (Kyé7e) and Me* (Harvey and Hulko 2013). Whereas *The Mind Thief* (Framst and Harvey 2015) is replete with biomedical information on Alzheimer's disease and strategies for maintaining brain health, the Tahltan language does not appear at all in this forty-four-page novel. Nor does a map of the nation's territory. In contrast, *A Good Day with Grandma (Kyé7e) and Me* includes more Secwepemc knowledge than biomedical, focuses on strengths rather than deficits, integrates the Secwepemcstín language throughout, and names the seventeen communities in Secwepemc territory. Though both of these books are dementia knowledge translation tools developed in consultation with BC First Nations, featuring illustrations by the same First Nation artist, they are nation-specific and distinctly different from one another. However, this is not to say that either the process of developing the books or the books themselves would not be useful to other First Nations or communities.

There is much that a comparatively young society such as Canada can learn from the more mature Secwepemc Nation, not the least of which is valuing older people and demonstrating a deep compassion and respect for them. Our teaching tools could not only strengthen Secwepemc worldviews within and across Indigenous communities, but could also influence broader society. For example, educators in Canadian public schools could use them to introduce students to dementia – and the importance of maintaining their own brain health – in a loving and respectful way that promotes compassion and inclusion, rather than fear and isolation.

There remains space for the co-creation and/or sharing of Indigenous ways of understanding and responding to memory loss in later life, not only in other settler nations, but also with First Nations, Métis, and Inuit peoples throughout Canada. Future research could assess the impact of teaching tools such as these on relations between Elders and young people and on understandings of memory loss and aging. This could be done through the schools or the communities. For example, it would be interesting to track the conversations started within families and communities by reading the storybook and/or watching the video together. Researching the use of the tools – in their intended and unintended ways – would be a fruitful area to explore. KTE should be an integral part of future dementia research with Indigenous people, building on Stories of Our Past.

When researchers are doing collaborative work with Indigenous people in Canada, and the project is grounded in Indigenous worldviews, the research process must also be rooted in Indigenous (nation-specific) traditions and values (Kovach 2010; Wilson 2008). It is customary for visitors to present a gift to the hosting chief as payment for safe passage on the traditional territory and as an indication of the good intentions of the guests. Gifting to a storyteller is also customary to recognize their skills and time spent with the guests. Thus, it is important that researchers gift their Indigenous partners for their participation. Overarching this gifting process is the idea of stewardship, which involves considering the impact of one's actions on future generations; some Indigenous people plan with the next seven generations in mind.

Collaborative research such as this goes beyond the recognition of participants as co-authors in publications to encouraging researchers to leave a lasting legacy that will benefit future generations of Indigenous people. Best practices for researchers would be to honour the Indigenous people with whom they work by undertaking studies that reflect local Indigenous customs and values, ensuring that reciprocity is embedded in the planning stage and that the final gift is meaningful, impactful, and sustainable.

Acknowledgments

Stories of Our Past was funded by the Canadian Dementia Knowledge Translation Network and the Alzheimer Society of Canada. The CSDC project was funded by the Michael Smith Foundation for Health Research through the BC Nursing Research Initiative. We thank all the CSDC team members, especially the Elder advisers and the participating communities, without whom the project would not have been possible.

Notes

1   The responses to questionnaires have been edited only to ensure accurate spelling of community names.

2   The Secwepemc people traditionally see memory loss in later life as part of going through the full circle of life. A person moves around the circle from the spiritual realm, to birth, to youth, to adulthood, to old age, with the final phase representing a return to the spiritual realm (see Hulko et al. 2010).

3   For the Thompson Rivers University website, visit Thompson Rivers University, "Elder Stories Reconnect Generations," December 20, 2103, http://inside.tru.ca/2013/12/20/elder-stories.

References

Alzheimer Society of Canada. 2014. "Helping Children." http://www.alzheimer.ca/en/Living-with-dementia/Staying-connected/Helping-children.

Archibald, Jo-Ann. 2008. *Indigenous Storywork: Educating the Heart, Mind, Body, and Spirit.* Vancouver: UBC Press.

Banner Alzheimer's Institute. 2010. *Alzheimer's Disease: Stories from Caregivers.* Video produced for the Banner Alzheimer's Institute Native American Outreach Program. https://www.youtube.com/watch?v=I2BITdZgRr0.

Basting, Anne Davis. 2009. *Forget Memory: Creating Better Lives for People with Dementia.*

Baltimore: Johns Hopkins University Press.

Battiste, Marie. 2013. *Decolonizing Education: Nourishing the Learning Spirit.* Saskatoon: Purich.

Carter, Leona. 2012, February 11. "Kehteyak (Meaning 'the Old Ones' in Cree): Functional Roles of Older Aboriginal People in Aboriginal Communities." In *Elder Protocol and Guidelines,* Council on Aboriginal Initiatives, 9–12. Edmonton: Council on Aboriginal Initiatives, University of Alberta. https://cloudfront.ualberta.ca/-/media/ualberta/office-of-the-provost-and-vice-president/indigenous-files/elder-protocol.pdf.

Chow, Tiffany, and Gail Elliot. 2012. "Frank and Tess – Detectives! A Children's Activity Book about Frontotemporal Degeneration (FTD)." http://research.baycrest.org/files/Frank-and-Tess-Detectives-.pdf.

Crowe-Salazar, Noela. 2007. "Exploring the Experiences of an Elder, a Psychologist and a Psychiatrist: How Can Traditional Practices and Healers Complement Existing Practices in Mental Health?" *First Peoples Child and Family Review* 3 (4): 83–95.

Framst, Louise S., and Karlene Harvey. 2015. "The Mind Thief: A Kid's Guide to Alzheimer's Disease." http://med-fom-neuroethics.sites.olt.ubc.ca/files/2015/08/GTP-The-Mind-Thief-s1.pdf.

Gerdner, Paula. 2008. *Grandfather's Story Cloth.* New York: Shen's Books.

Harvey, Karlene, with Wendy Hulko. 2013. *A Good Day with Grandma (Kyé7e) and Me.* Kamloops, BC: Thompson Rivers University. https://www.tru.ca/blobs/whulko/childrens-book-for-web.pdf.

Hulko, Wendy. 2009. "From 'Not a Big Deal' to 'Hellish': Experiences of Older People with Dementia." *Journal of Aging Studies* 23 (3): 131–44. DOI:10.1016/j.jaging.2007.11.002.

Hulko, Wendy, Evelyn Camille, Elizabeth Antifeau, Michael Arnouse, N. Bachynksi, and D. Taylor. 2010. "Views of First Nation Elders on Memory Loss and Memory Care in Later Life." *Journal of Cross-Cultural Gerontology* 25 (4): 317–42. DOI:10.1007/s10823-010-9123-9.

Hulko, Wendy, D. Wilson, S. Mahara, J. Williams, E. Patrick Moller, C. DeRose, G. Campbell McArthur, L. Michel-Evans, and A. Parkscott. 2014, October. "Culturally Safe Dementia Care: Building Nursing Capacity to Care for First Nation Elders with Memory Loss." Workshop presentation at International Network of Indigenous Health Knowledge and Development and Network Environments for Aboriginal Health Research conference, Winnipeg.

Illes, Judy, N. Chahal, and B. Lynn Beattie. 2011. "A Landscape for Training in Dementia Knowledge Translation (DKT)." *Gerontology and Geriatrics* 32 (3): 260–72.

Jacobs Altman, Linda, and Larry Johnson. 2002. *Singing with Momma Lou.* New York: Lee and Low Books.

Kakugawa, Frances H., and Melissa DeSica. 2007. *Wordsworth Dances the Waltz.* Honolulu: Watermark.

Kovach, Margaret. 2010. *Indigenous Methodologies: Characteristics, Conversations, and Contexts.* Toronto: University of Toronto Press.

Loyie, L., and C. Brissenden. 2012. *The Gathering Tree*. Penticton, BC: Theytus Books.

Mack, Trevor, with Wendy Hulko. 2013. *Remembering Our Way Forward: Dementia from a Secwepemc Perspective*. Video produced for Stories of Our Past: A Dementia Knowledge Translation Project between First Nations Elders and Children. Kamloops, BC: Thompson Rivers University.

Manthorpe, Jill. 2005. "A Child's Eye View: Dementia in Children's Literature." *British Journal of Social Work* 35: 305–20.

Mehl-Madrona, Lewis. 2009. "What Traditional Indigenous Elders Say about Cross-Cultural Mental Health Training." *Explore* 5 (1): 20–29. DOI:10.1016/j.explore.2008.10.003.

Nichols, Katherine, and Tiffany Chow. 2011. "When Dementia Is in the House." http://lifeandminds.ca/whendementiaisinthehouse.

Pace, Jessica E., Lisa Boesch, and Kristen Jacklin. 2010, August 30. "National Aboriginal Alzheimer's Disease and Related Dementias (ADRD) Research Network Meeting: April 15 and 16, 2010 Northern Ontario School of Medicine, Meeting Report." https://docs.wixstatic.com/ugd/6e29de_1455eea44f02419b942721debc8585e5.pdf.

Rosenbluth, Roz. 2005. *Getting to Know Ruben Plotnick*. Brooklyn: Flashlight Press.

Shepherd, Jessica. 2014. *Grandma*. Swindon, UK: Child's Play (International).

Smith, Peter, dir. N.d. *Love in the Time of Dementia*. Tiwi, AU: Carpentaria Disability Services and isee-ilearn, Film. https://www.youtube.com/watch?v=hKfGfbn6rtw.

Statistics Canada. 2013. "Individual Internet Use and E-Commerce, 2012." *The Daily*. http://www.statcan.gc.ca/daily-quotidien/131028/dq131028a-eng.htm.

Varcoe, Colleen, Helen Brown, Betty Calam, M. Buchanan, and V. Newman. 2011. "Capacity Building Is a Two-Way Street: Learning from Doing Research in Aboriginal Communities." In *Feminist Community Research: Case Studies and Methodologies,* ed. G. Creese and W. Frisby, 210–31. Vancouver: UBC Press.

Wilson, Shawn. 2008. *Research Is Ceremony: Indigenous Research Methods*. Halifax: Fernwood.

CONCLUSION

Wendy Hulko, Jean E. Balestrery,
and Danielle Wilson

AS DEMONSTRATED BY the research presented in this book, dementia is more than a biological diagnosis for Indigenous people. Elders with dementia have a cascading effect on the entire social fabric of their community because they continue to be embedded within families and communities. As the few remaining cultural knowledge keepers age, a certain number will develop dementia, and thus health care workers must modify and update their care of Elders. However, Indigenous people are resilient and are developing strengths-based approaches to improve health outcomes through preventing memory loss and caring for Elders with dementia in a culturally safe manner. Strengths-based approaches featured in this book include using storytelling to share knowledge, viewing dementia as a part of the life cycle and a return to childhood (the spirit realm) as natural, involving children and youth in the care of Elders, designing interventions based on Indigenous knowledge, and having allies play an active role in challenging colonization.

It is quite possible that the causal connections between colonization and dementia, as detailed in the Indigenous Syndemic Dementia Model for the United States, could also be observed in other settler colonial states such as Canada, New Zealand, and Australia. Understanding the cascading health effects of historical trauma is paramount for the provision of culturally safe care and for the promotion of activities to maintain brain health. Indigenous people must inform and ideally lead these activities, with the support of settler allies in the spirit of collaboration and reconciliation.

Dementia rates for Indigenous people are predicted to increase dramatically over the next decades. In Canada, for example, the rates will be nearly twice those of the non-Indigenous population by 2031; if risk factors were taken into consideration, the expected dementia rates would be even higher among the Indigenous population. Thus, health promotion activities are ever more important, as is a call to action on the social determinants of Indigenous people's health to influence the projected rates of dementia. This could include supporting or reviving IndigenACTION, a physical activity initiative for Indigenous people that was promoted during the 2010 Winter Olympics in Vancouver (IndigenACTION 2012). Returning to a traditional diet, which includes brain-healthy foods such as salmon and blueberries, could also be encouraged.

Indigenous people still face discrimination and adverse reactions to such calls to action, however. This can be seen in the media, where Indigenous people with dementia are portrayed with a lack of empathy and an emphasis on criminalization. Print and social media will play an important role in advocacy efforts, including informing non-Indigenous people about the health inequities of Indigenous people and the need for collaborative action.

As illustrated by our exploration of Indigenous perspectives on care and prevention, individual, family, and community views on memory loss in later life are indeed shaped by socioeconomic and geopolitical contexts, as are the experiences of people with dementia and those who care for them. Thus, large-scale social processes such as colonization and decolonization have clearly affected the understanding and experience of dementia for Indigenous people across Turtle Island and other continents. There is a need for greater awareness of dementia in First Nations communities, and the support for caregivers should not only be increased, but also made more culturally relevant and safe.

Traditional knowledge can and should be applied to the care of Elders who are experiencing memory loss. This could include the use of the medicine wheel with Anishinaabe people or the adoption of whānau-based care for Māori, as well as other approaches derived from Indigenous knowledge. It is essential to develop and preserve Indigenous models of care and treatment, as an appreciation of history and a focus on healing is integral to these models. In an era of reconciliation, this needs to be a priority to ensure that dementia care is culturally relevant and safe. It must be designed and delivered to meet more than the physical needs of Elders: it must be holistic, in that it also meets their emotional, mental, and spiritual needs. It should be compassionate and based on the Indigenous principles of reciprocity, wisdom, and trust.

Although Indigenous people's views and experiences share similarities, there are also significant differences. As a result, we need to avoid a pan-Indigenous approach (see Kovach 2009) while at the same time engaging in "cultural humility" (Foronda et al. 2016). Further research and the translation of research findings into improved care – at the level of both policy and practice – should be led by collaborative teams composed of Indigenous people and settler allies. These teams must be knowledgeable about and accountable to the community or First Nation that is participating in the study. Once culturally specific local information has been gathered and analyzed, and there is a solid understanding of and appreciation for that community or nation's approach to dementia, connections can be made across communities, nations, and continents. We are all trying to support a strong Indigenous movement to reclaim health and eliminate health disparities for Indigenous peoples.

Elders' voices, prominently featured in the research and teaching stories that appear in this book, showcase the experiences and wisdom of Elders from across Turtle Island. This work is the result of collaborative research by Indigenous and non-Indigenous individuals who are committed to doing research "in a good way" (Ball and Janysk 2008) and that "will mean something" for participants (Jacklin and Kinoshameg 2008). This approach makes a difference, not only to the process for everyone involved, but also to the knowledge created and to decolonization efforts in general. These narratives demonstrate the significant role that storytelling continues to play in Indigenous communities as a method of knowledge translation and exchange (KTE). Further, storytelling and reminiscence are important means of preserving the memories of Elders and of responding to memory loss in a culturally safe way. Integrating experiential knowledge and reflecting traditional means of sharing knowledge, such as teaching stories, honours the contributions of Elders to the research featured in this book and enhances the learning to be gained by our readers.

The framework of KTE is both conceptual and practical. Teaching and learning each inform the other. KTE refers to mutual exchange and access to resources for mutual benefit across cultural differences and contexts. It is predicated on processes of "mutual empowerment, where Aboriginal communities and individuals at risk can take equal part in the solutions" (Brascoupé and Waters 2009, 17). Consequently, there are risks and rewards for all involved, such as mutual accountability and mutual benefit. KTE promotes holistic healing and community partnership, and it has the potential to heal cultural anomie (Brascoupé and Waters 2009).

We recommend that future studies with Indigenous people make use of Indigenous research methodologies (IRM) and that they incorporate KTE into their design. KTE offers mutual benefits in diverse contexts, including Indigenous communities and academic institutions. Acknowledging and increasing awareness of history can and should be a motivator for communities to engage with researchers. At the same time, academic institutions need to be more accepting of IRM by supporting research proposals, ethical review applications, publications, and tenure applications that involve it. Indigenous scholars and settler allies are at the forefront of IRM, particularly in Canada, and their leadership should be respected and acknowledged. Ultimately, research based on IRM and the application of findings to practice can generate dementia care that goes beyond physiological health and takes into consideration mental, emotional, and spiritual health.

As shown in the chapters on the application of theory and knowledge to practice, KTE presents creative avenues for increasing understanding. Among Indigenous communities, it necessarily involves Elders because they are viewed as the bearers of cultural tradition and wisdom. As evidenced in many of the preceding chapters and the teaching story interludes, the voices and views of Indigenous Elders are prominent.

Elders emphasize the importance of both individual and collective memory in the context of colonization, decolonization, and reconciliation. Yet, most essentially, they identify a dialectical tension that exists in processes of detection and diagnosis of memory loss. This tension occurs between some Indigenous people who do not wish to recall past memories – and who may express a conscious memory loss – and those who enjoy reminiscing about the past. Elders caution that automatic assumptions should not be embedded in any health or social service intervention and encourage the development of practical tools that can benefit Indigenous communities. Such tools can strengthen intergenerational relationships and honour traditional perspectives.

The insights offered by our contributors enrich interdisciplinary perspectives on dementia and apply across socioeconomic and geopolitical contexts. This book moves beyond the dominant narrative of dementia, which is often marked by negativity (Beard 2016; Hulko 2009), to emphasize a strengths-based approach that is consistent with Indigenous values and traditions. Thus, it is reflective of a critical tradition in dementia studies that began with critiques of the biomedicalization of dementia (Lyman 1989) and the social construction of Alzheimer's disease (Gubrium 1986) and has led to calls for a social citizenship approach (Bartlett and O'Connor 2010). These seek to promote a more hopeful, complex, comprehensive, and critical perspective on persons living with dementia (Bartlett and O'Connor 2010, 7). This book contributes to these efforts to challenge the dominant narrative, thereby shifting representations of people who have dementia and the communities in which they live.

The innovative research featured in these pages has numerous implications for policy, practice, and research, all of which are interrelated. Articulating such implications and then reshaping practice and policy should involve many stakeholders, including researchers, practitioners, policy makers, and community members. This reshaping will affect health care systems and academic institutions alike, particularly their organizational structures and decision-making processes, and the approaches to practice and research that are favoured or valued in these socioeconomic and geopolitical contexts.

Practitioners first need to appreciate that dementia is relevant to Indigenous communities because its prevalence is higher than previously thought and is expected to increase. Furthermore, communities are asking for assistance. If practitioners support communities to address Indigenous social determinants of health (see Greenwood et al. 2015), the expected increase in the incidence of dementia could be turned around. The emerging new science of epigenetics (see Pember 2017) affirms Indigenous principles of relationality and interconnectedness and conceptions of health as physical, mental, emotional, *and* spiritual. As Mary Annette Pember (2017) points out, historical trauma "can be seen as a contributing cause in the development of illnesses such as PTSD, depression and type 2 diabetes," a statement that is supported by the Indigenous Syndemic Dementia Model presented in this book. Further, being aware of historical trauma and appreciating that the past plays an ongoing and significant role in the present are key for health and social care practitioners. Thus, organizations can better support their staff by offering trauma-informed training and enabling connections with Elders and other community resource people. Drawing on traditional knowledge when working with Elders living with dementia and their family and community will ensure the provision of more culturally safe practice.

Organizational leaders are instrumental in transforming the policies and procedures that guide the delivery of memory care services. In supporting collaboration with Indigenous people and communities to address memory loss and dementia, organizational leaders must understand that "the pervasive and harmful impact of traumatic events on individuals, families and communities and the unintended but similarly widespread re-traumatizing of individuals within our public institutions and service systems, makes it necessary to rethink doing 'business as usual'" (SAMHSA 2014, 2). Currently, "there is an increasing focus on the impact of trauma and how service systems may help to resolve or exacerbate trauma-related issues" (SAMHSA 2014, 2). This focus has resulted in emerging interventions, particularly in the United States and Canada, such as the adoption by health care systems of a trauma-informed approach and a shift from hospital and residential care services to those based in the community. Further, implementing KTE in research reflects a trauma-informed approach that can foster a more trusting relationship with researchers and lead to improved health care outcomes for Indigenous people and communities.

Any national or provincial policies on dementia that are developed and/ or promoted by settler colonial states should acknowledge the unique context of Indigenous peoples and make a concerted effort to avoid pan-indigenizing. The National Strategy for Alzheimer's Disease and Other Dementias Act (Government of Canada 2017) does not refer to Indigenous peoples and emphasizes the "burden" caused by persons "suffering from dementia." This act is another clear example of a biomedical or clinical approach to dementia rather than a holistic or strengths-based one that would be more consistent with Indigenous worldviews. It requires the establishment of an advisory board whose fifteen members are to be appointed by the minister of health. We hope that the diversity of persons living with dementia and their families and communities will be reflected in the composition of this board and in its work. Similarly, we encourage the other settler colonial states to apply the principles of inclusion and representation to their policy development and implementation work related to dementia.

To avoid pan-indigenizing, community- or nation-specific differences must be understood and respected. At the level of the health system, policy development and revision should include consideration of trauma and should acknowledge community- and nation-specific traditions. For example, end-of-life ceremonies vary from family to community to nation. They can include bathing rituals for the person who has passed, burning ceremonies with sacred fire or smudging, and even Christian traditions such as last rites. Thus, residential care facilities should develop their policies through local consultation to reflect and respect the traditions and strengths of the communities and nations that they serve.

The insights garnered about Indigenous people and dementia, many of which are showcased in this book, offer numerous avenues for researchers to explore in collaboration with Indigenous communities. They should include and respect traditional knowledge, particularly those who use IRM. To date, the perspectives and concerns of care providers, both formal and informal, have been over-emphasized, and the views and experiences of people living with dementia have been neglected. Thus, future research should include and respect Elders who are experiencing memory loss and/or receiving memory care. This book has provided guidance to assist with such efforts.

Although this book focuses on Indigenous people, other marginalized persons and equity-seeking groups will benefit from the knowledge collected herein. In moving past the dominant narrative of dementia, the book is relevant to all those who struggle against health inequities and seek a more socially just world. It also contributes to interdisciplinary conversations at the intersection of evidence-based practice and cultural competence (Gone 2015), as well as those on cultural safety and cultural humility, all of which are highly relevant in an increasingly diverse world. Being able to build a bridge between the past and the present is essential for Indigenous people, who are experiencing the relatively new phenomenon of dementia. Settler allies who work with them need to respect the bridging that is actively occurring and display cultural humility. Although this book speaks specifically to memory loss and dementia care, many of the principles and approaches that it discusses will be useful to Indigenous people who are tackling other health inequities beyond dementia.

References

Ball, Jessica, and P. Janysk. 2008. "Enacting Research Ethics in Partnerships with Indigenous Communities in Canada: 'Do It in a Good Way.'" *Journal of Empirical Research on Human Research Ethics* 3 (2): 33–51.

Bartlett, Ruth, and Deborah O'Connor. 2010. *Broadening the Dementia Debate: Towards Social Citizenship.* Bristol: Policy Press.

Beard, Renée L. 2016. *Living with Alzheimer's: Managing Memory Loss, Identity and Illness.* New York: New York University Press.

Brascoupé, Simon, and Catherine Waters. 2009. "Cultural Safety, Exploring the Applicability of the Concept of Cultural Safety to Aboriginal Health and Community Wellness." *International Journal of Aboriginal Health* 5 (2): 6–41.

Foronda, Cynthia, Diana-Lyn Baptiste, Maren M. Reinholdt, and Kevin Ousman. 2016. "Cultural Humility: A Concept Analysis." *Journal of Transcultural Nursing* 27 (3): 210–17. DOI:10.1177/1043659615592677.

Gone, J. 2015. "Reconciling Evidence-Based Practice and Cultural Competence in Mental Health Services: Introduction to a Special Issue." *Transcultural Psychiatry* 52 (2): 139–49.

Government of Canada. 2017. *National Strategy for Alzheimer's Disease and Other Dementias Act,* S.C. 2017, c. 19. http://laws-lois.justice.gc.ca/eng/AnnualStatutes /2017_19/page-1.html.

Greenwood, M., S. de Leeuw, N.M. Lindsay, and C. Reading. 2015. *Determinants of Indigenous Peoples' Health in Canada: Beyond the Social.* Toronto: Canadian Scholars' Press.

Gubrium, Jaber. 1986. *Oldtimers and Alzheimer's: The Descriptive Organization of Senility.* Greenwich, CT: JAI Press.

Hulko, Wendy. 2009. "From 'Not a Big Deal' to 'Hellish': Experiences of Older People with Dementia." *Journal of Aging Studies* 23 (3): 131–44. DOI:10.1016/j.jaging .2007.11.002.

IndigenACTION. 2012. "Phase One: Roundtable Report." http://www.afn.ca/uploads/ files/indigenaction/indigenactionroundtablereport.pdf.

Jacklin, Kristen, and P. Kinoshameg. 2008. "Developing a Participatory Aboriginal Health Research Project: 'Only if It's Going to Mean Something.'" *Journal of Empirical Research in Human Research Ethics* 3 (2): 53–68.

Kovach, Margaret. 2009. *Indigenous Methodologies: Characteristics, Conversations, and Contexts.* Toronto: University of Toronto Press.

Lyman, Karen. 1989. "Bringing the Social Back In: A Critique of the Biomedicalization of Dementia." *Gerontologist* 29 (5): 597–605.

Pember, Mary Annette. 2017, October 3. "Trauma May Be Woven into DNA of Native Americans." *Indian Country Today.* First published May 28, 2015. https://newsmaven. io/indiancountrytoday/archive/trauma-may-be-woven-into-dna-of-native -americans-CbiAxpzaroWkMALhjrcGVQ/.

SAMHSA (Substance Abuse and Mental Health Services Administration). 2014. *SAMHSA's Concept of Trauma and Guidance for a Trauma-Informed Approach.* HHS Publication No. (SMA) 14-4884. Rockville, MD: SAMHSA.

ACKNOWLEDGMENTS

FIRST, WE WOULD LIKE to thank our funders. The 2013 roundtable forum on indigeneity and dementia at Thompson Rivers University (TRU), to which most of the chapter authors contributed and which led to this edited book, was made possible through a $20,000 Canadian Institutes of Health Research (CIHR) meeting grant awarded to Wendy Hulko and Tracy Christianson. We gratefully acknowledge Laura Michel-Evans and Jessica Kent for their assistance with the roundtable forum and the International Indigenous Dementia Research Network for creating a platform to exchange knowledge and foster collaborative work, such as this book.

The CIHR grant, together with the Culturally Safe Dementia Care (CSDC) research grant of $217,300 that Wendy Hulko and the CSDC team received from the Michael Smith Foundation for Health Research, enabled us to hire undergraduate research assistant Anna Parkscott, whom the editors sincerely thank for her contributions to this collection. The $1,000 Wendy received from TRU for the 2019 Undergraduate Research Mentor Award allowed us to hire Bachelor of Social Work student Robert Long and Bachelor of Social Work alumna Emma Peppall-Schultz to work on the index, and we are extremely grateful for their contributions and flexibility.

We would also like to thank TRU, our colleagues, and our families for recognizing the significance of this book and for encouraging its completion. Chris Walmsley (TRU) in particular offered important insights on book publishing and working with contributing authors. Kukstemc to TRU and to Dean Airini of the Faculty of Education and Social Work for assistance with publication costs ($5,000) and advocacy for Indigenous peoples.

We are grateful to Darcy Cullen, Katrina Petrik, and the other editorial staff at UBC Press, who were responsive and enthusiastic throughout this process, and to the anonymous peer reviewers, who provided helpful suggestions. Any errors or omissions are our own, however.

Lastly, we thank all the contributors for joining us in this effort to increase respect for Indigenous knowledge and to broaden the landscape of dementia research, and for making this book such an interesting and dynamic collection.

CONTRIBUTORS

JEAN E. BALESTRERY, PhD social work and anthropology (University of Michigan), MA anthropology (University of Michigan), MSW (University of Washington), BA (Brown University), is a licensed independent practitioner and former assistant clinical professor in the Department of Sociology and Social Work, Northern Arizona University, Flagstaff. Dr. Balestrery conducts research in health and aging, and has presented internationally. She is a Spirit of EAGLES Hampton Faculty Fellow addressing American Indian and Alaska Native (AIAN) cancer disparities and was selected as scholar-participant for the Translational Health Disparities course with National Institutes of Health, Bethesda, Maryland. Dr. Balestrery served on the Council of Sexual Orientation, Gender Identity and Expression with the Council on Social Work Education. She can be reached at jbalestrery@gmail.com.

MELISSA BLIND is Cree and Ukrainian, and a member of Gordon's First Nation, in the Treaty 4 area. She has a PhD in American Indian studies from the University of Arizona and holds a BA (Honours) and a MA in Indigenous studies from First Nations University of Canada in conjunction with the University of Regina. Dr. Blind is a senior research associate for the Memory Keepers Medical Discovery Team (MK MDT) at the University of Minnesota Medical School, Duluth. Prior to joining the MK MDT, she was a research associate with the Centre for Rural and Northern Health Research, working closely with Dr. Kristen Jacklin on the Canadian Consortium on Neurodegeneration in Aging Team 20 Indigenous dementia projects in Ontario. Her research interests include Indigenous understandings of health and well-being (including health disparities), Indigenous understandings of neurological conditions such as dementia and Alzheimer's Disease, issues surrounding identity, and oral narratives.

CARRIE BOURASSA is a professor of Indigenous health in the College of Medicine, Department of Community Health and Epidemiology at the University of Saskatchewan. Dr. Bourassa spent over fifteen years as a professor of Indigenous health studies in the Department of Indigenous Health, Education and Social Work at the First Nations University of Canada in Regina. She is the scientific director of the Institute of Indigenous Peoples' Health (IIPH) in the Canadian Institutes of Health Research. Through IIPH, she leads the advancement of a national health research agenda to improve and promote the health of First Nations, Inuit, and Métis peoples in Canada. Dr. Bourassa is a member of the College of New Scholars, Artists and Scientists of the Royal Society of Canada and a public member of the Royal College Council of the Royal College of Physicians and Surgeons of Canada. Her research interests include the impacts of colonization on the health of First Nations and Métis people, creating culturally safe care in health service delivery, Indigenous community-based health research methodology, HIV/AIDS research among Indigenous people, end-of-life care among Indigenous people, dementia among Indigenous people, and Indigenous women's health. Dr. Bourassa is Métis and belongs to the Riel Métis Council of Regina Inc. (RMCR, Local #34).

GWENDYLINE CAMPBELL MCARTHUR, RPN (non-practising), RN, BScN – MH Spec., MN, is of Ojibwe/Saulteaux Métis and Ukrainian ancestry. She recently retired from full-time nursing to work in independent practice. Gwen's work as a psychiatric mental health nurse spanned five decades, guided by Indigenous Elders and other spiritual leaders. Now living in British Columbia, where she raised her two sons, she is honoured to work with Thompson Rivers University and the research team that included Secwepemc Elders. Gwen has published on psychiatric mental health nursing and Indigenous community health nursing in several important nursing textbooks.

LINDA D. CARSON was an associate professor in the College of Public Health at the University of Oklahoma and center coordinator for the American Indian Diabetes Prevention Center, funded by the National Institutes of Health – National Institute on Minority Health and Disparities. She is now a consultant with the International Association for Indigenous Aging. She holds degrees in nursing, public health epidemiology, and aging studies. Her interdisciplinary research focuses on cross-cultural health communications surrounding diabetes and dementia. Dr. Carson has examined diverse cultural models of diabetes in American Indian elder populations, health care delivery models among tribal health care providers, the cultural construction of dementia among American Indian caregivers, and the delivery of health communications regarding bioterrorism to culturally diverse populations. At the national level, her grant review service includes the Centers for Disease Control and Prevention (CDC) Special Emphasis Panel: Surveillance, Natural History, Quality of Care and Outcomes of Diabetes Mellitus with Onset in Childhood and Adolescence, the CDC Special Diabetes Panel Community-Directed Grant Program, and the Indian Health Service. In 2012, Dr. Carson was inducted into the national Delta Omega Honorary Society in Public Health. (Dr. Carson's work has also been published under the name L. Carson Henderson.)

CECILIA DICK DEROSE is a member of Esketemc First Nation. Described as a pillar in preserving her language and culture, Cecilia teaches ethnobotany and the Secwepemcstín language at the Williams Lake campus of Thompson Rivers University. She works with both the Elders College in Williams Lake and a local Aboriginal Head Start program. Cecilia was an Elder adviser to the Culturally Safe Dementia Care research project; she was involved in the education sessions with the nurse participants, and with the sharing of the research findings. DeRose was given an Indspire Award in March 2018 in recognition of her leadership in preserving Secwepemc language and culture, including tanning, beading, and medicinal plants.

J. NEIL HENDERSON is a professor of family medicine and biobehavioral health and executive director of the Memory Keepers Medical Discovery Team on Health Equity at the University of Minnesota Medical School, Duluth. He was formerly the Edith K. Gaylord Presidential Professor at the University of Oklahoma Health Sciences Center, Department of Health Promotion Sciences, and director of the American Indian Diabetes Prevention Center in the College of Public Health, Oklahoma City. He is Oklahoma Choctaw. His research focuses on aging issues of American Indian people. He has undertaken biocultural research on Alzheimer's disease in American Indian tribes, developed Alzheimer's support groups in African American and Spanish-speaking populations, and conducted geriatric health care education for American Indian providers across the United States. The author of many articles, he is co-author of *Social and*

Behavioral Foundations of Public Health (2001) and is the principal author of *The Savvy Caregiver for Indian Country* (2013).

WENDY HULKO, third-generation Canadian of Scottish, Swedish, and Finnish ancestry, is an associate professor and Bachelor of Social Work program coordinator in the Faculty of Education and Social Work at Thompson Rivers University. Wendy holds a BA (Hons.) in sociology and Spanish (Trent University), a MSW (University of Toronto), and a PhD in sociology and social policy (University of Stirling). She has worked in the field of aging for over twenty-five years, including residential care nursing, hospital social work, and government policy. Wendy conducts interdisciplinary research on aging and health in collaboration with Interior Health (British Columbia) and equity-seeking groups, including Secwepemc Nation Elders. In July 2013, she co-hosted a Canadian Institutes of Health Research–funded roundtable forum on indigeneity and dementia at TRU. Dr. Hulko has published extensively in peer-reviewed journals and edited books and was the recipient of the 2016 Thompson Rivers University Excellence in Scholarship Award and the 2019 TRU Undergraduate Research Mentor Award.

KRISTEN JACKLIN, PhD, is a professor in the Department of Family Medicine and Biobehavioral Health and associate director of the Memory Keepers Medical Discovery Team on Health Equity at the University of Minnesota Medical School, Duluth. Dr. Jacklin is a medical anthropologist with an extensive background in community-based Indigenous health research and health equity. Her research focuses on chronic disease care for Indigenous peoples, including investigations concerning aging, cognitive health and dementia, diabetes, and Indigenous health/medical education. Dr. Jacklin holds research funding related to the study of dementia from several sources including the National Institutes of Health and the Canadian Institutes of Health Research. Dr. Jacklin is the founder of the International Indigenous Dementia Research Network and the Indigenous Cognition Awareness and Aging Awareness Research Exchange (I-CAARE.ca).

JESSICA KENT is a settler of Western European heritage. She was raised in Sechelt Nation territory on British Columbia's Sunshine Coast. She currently lives in Armstrong, British Columbia, near the intersection of Secwepemc and Syilx territories, with her husband and son. Jessica worked on the Stories of Our Past project as a practicum student and then as a research assistant while completing her Bachelor of Social Work at Thompson Rivers University. She also has an advanced diploma in independent digital film-making and a certificate in Indigenous studies. Since completing her social work degree, Jessica has been doing community engagement work with one of the Secwepemc Nation's health centres.

MERE KĒPA undertook the care and responsibility for her late father, Tiakiriri Kēpa Kukupa. On behalf of her extended family and tribes, she is active in writing submissions to local, regional, and national government agencies. She is a sociocultural innovator who works to inspire a new vision of later life. She was a senior Māori academic on the project "Life and Living in Advanced Age: A Cohort Study in New Zealand." Presently, she is involved in "Nga Kaumatua, o Matou Taonga: Supporting Kaumatua Health in a Changing World – A Feasibility Study in Te Tai Tokerau."

KAMA KING is a research associate at the American Indian Diabetes Prevention Center (AIDPC), housed in the College of Public Health at the University of Oklahoma Health Sciences Center. She is currently assisting in research at the AIDPC that focuses on relieving health disparities among American Indian populations, through understanding of the biocultural factors that influence the treatment and prevention of diabetes. Her current research includes parental distress associated with caring for a diabetic child, health beliefs about prevention of diabetes among pregnant women, and cultural barriers to successful treatment of diabetes. She is also an adjunct professor at the University of Central Oklahoma.

SUZANNE MACLEOD is a fourth-generation settler who is grateful to live in Victoria, British Columbia, with her partner and two daughters on the territory of the Chilcowitch people, who were ancestors to the present-day Songhees First Nation. She is a social worker in a long-term-care home for people who have dementia. During her master's in social work studies, she thought about dominant dementia discourses in health care policy in a neoliberal context; Indigenous approaches to dementia and decolonizing dementia care; dementia and resistance through international self-advocacy and localized poetics; and local eating and social policy – namely, the Seasonal Agricultural Worker Program – as racialized practice. She also enjoys riding her bike and growing veggies.

M. STAR MAHARA is an associate professor in the School of Nursing at Thompson Rivers University. Over the past fifteen years, she has worked in partnership with many individuals and groups to improve the post-secondary experience of Indigenous nursing students. She has also been active in initiatives to integrate critical cultural perspectives in nursing education and practice. She is a past recipient of the Canadian Association of Schools of Nursing Award for Excellence in Nursing Education. Her teaching and research interests include nursing education, cultural safety and culturally safe dementia care, and Indigenous new graduate nurse transitions and career planning.

ROD MCCORMICK is Kanienkehaka (Mohawk) and a professor and British Columbia Innovation Council research chair in Aboriginal health in the Faculty of Education and Social Work at Thompson Rivers University (TRU) in Kamloops, British Columbia. One reason for his move to TRU in 2013 was because it is in the home territory of his partner and three of their children, who are members of the Tk'emlups te Secwepemc (Shuswap Nation). For almost twenty years, Rod worked as an Indigenous health researcher and professor in counselling psychology at the University of British Columbia (UBC) before moving to TRU. During a thirteen-year period while at UBC, he led three different provincial networks in Indigenous health research in British Columbia.

SOPHIE "EQEELANA TUNGWENUK" NOTHSTINE was born at Cape Prince of Wales, Alaska. Named after her maternal great-aunt, she was raised very traditionally by her Inupiaq father, Louis Tungwenuk, and her mother, Adele Kuyuk. She has seven sisters and one brother. Her father, a subsistence hunter and reindeer herder, was a store keeper and leader of Wales. Sophie has a bachelor's degree in social work and three years of a master's in social work. For more than twenty years, she worked in Alaska as a drug/alcohol counsellor and social worker. She has her own Inupiaq dance group, Kingikmuit Dance Group, from the village of Wales. The dances were dormant for over fifty years because missionaries said they were evil and that all the white man's dances were evil too. So, dances were stopped completely until Richard Atuk, Sophie's son Gregory, and Sophie herself restarted them.

ERIC OLESON is the research supervisor for the Indigenous Community-Based Health Research Lab at the First Nations University of Canada. He has a bachelor's degree in political science and sociology and an economics certificate from the University of Regina, as well as a master's of public administration from the Johnson-Shoyama Graduate School of Public Policy. He has worked on many diverse projects pertaining to Indigenous health, HIV/AIDS, dementia, and intimate partner violence. Having worked on two Community-University Research Alliance grants and on multiple community-driven projects, Eric is an active ally in community-based participatory research.

JESSICA E. PACE obtained her PhD in the anthropology of health at McMaster University in 2013. She also completed an Alzheimer Society of Canada post-doctoral fellowship in the Department of Health, Aging and Society and the Gilbrea Centre for Studies in Aging at McMaster. Dr. Pace's community-based research focuses on perceptions of healthy aging, cultural understandings of dementia, approaches to care and treatment of people with dementia, and intergenerational relationships in Indigenous communities. Her research involves First Nations communities in Ontario and Southern Inuit communities in Labrador.

ESTELLA PATRICK MOLLER is from Nakazdli First Nations in Fort St. James. She is a fluent speaker of the Carrier language and loves sharing her knowledge of Carrier traditions, ceremonies, and women's ways. Estella is a strong believer in the healing properties of medicine and meditation and enjoys gathering medicines and making medicine bags. She is an Elder in Residence at Thompson Rivers University, and she has a passion for learning and sharing her knowledge and helping students focus on their personal development. She was an Elder adviser on the Culturally Safe Dementia Care project and played a key role throughout the research process, including the creation of the teaching stories.

KAREN PITAWANAKWAT is an Anishinaabe Kwe from the Wikwemikong Unceded Indian Reserve, Ontario. She has spent her life in Wikwemikong, leaving only to complete her nursing diploma at Cambrian College in 1994. She lives in Wikwemikong with her husband of twenty-five years. She is the mother of two children and grandmother to one. Karen belongs to the Thunder Bird Clan and is an Anishinaabemowin-language speaker. She has been nursing in local First Nations communities for twenty years, with a focus on homecare for older adults. She is currently the homecare co-ordinator for Nahndahweh Tchigeh Gamig (Wikwemikong Health Centre). Karen has been involved in community-based research projects concerning diabetes, dementia, and cancer since 2006 and has served continuously on the Wiwemikong Health Centre Diabetes Advisory Committee since 2005.

BARBARA PURVES is a speech-language pathologist and associate professor emerita in the School of Audiology and Speech Sciences at the University of British Columbia. Her clinical, teaching, and research activities have been mainly in the area of acquired communication disorders. Her research interests have focused on social aspects of living with such disorders, drawing on participatory design involving people with dementia or aphasia and their families to gain a deeper understanding of their perspectives and experiences. She has also co-designed and co-taught a graduate course for speech-language pathology and audiology students regarding culturally safe interaction and practice with people of Aboriginal heritage. A second-generation Canadian of predominantly English ancestry, Barbara spent most of her life on the shores of Burrard Inlet in the traditional territory of the Tsleil-Waututh Nation. She now lives in the Cowichan Valley, the traditional territory of the Quw'utsun' Nation.

KATE ROSS-HOPLEY is originally from Regina, Saskatchewan, where she completed her bachelor's degree in philosophy at the University of Regina. Currently, she is a student at the Mailman School of Public Health, Columbia University, where she is pursuing her master's of public health in the sociomedical sciences, with a certificate in health and human rights. She is also working as a research assistant at the First Nations University of Canada.

JENNIFER WALKER is a Haudenosaunee-settler health researcher and epidemiologist. She holds a PhD in epidemiology from the University of Calgary and a BSc in health studies from the University of Waterloo. Her research program focuses on Indigenous health and the use of health services across the life course, particularly among older adults. Dr. Walker is a principal investigator on a number of nationally funded research projects related to aging in Indigenous populations. She currently holds a Canada Research Chair in Indigenous Health and is an assistant professor at Laurentian University, School of Rural and Northern Health, and the Indigenous Lead and Scientist at the Institute for Clinical Evaluative Sciences.

WAYNE WARRY, PhD, is a professor in the Department of Family Medicine and Biobehavioral Health, and the director of Rural Health Initiatives on the Memory Keepers Medical Discovery Team on Health Equity at the University of Minnesota Medical School, Duluth. Dr. Warry is an applied medical anthropologist whose work involves a range of issues concerning health equity in rural and Indigenous communities in North America. His current research focuses on aging, diabetes, and dementia and on health systems access, quality of care, and cultural safety in health care. He is a member of Team 20 of the Canadian Consortium on Neurodegeneration in Aging and of the International Indigenous Dementia Research Network.

JEAN WILLIAM is a member of the T'exelcemc First Nation. She is an Elder, mentor, long-time Secwepemcstin language teacher in Williams Lake, British Columbia, and member of the Elders council of Three Corners Health Society in Williams Lake. Jean was an Elder adviser on the Culturally Safe Dementia Care project; she was involved in the education sessions with the nurse participants and the sharing of the research findings.

DANIELLE WILSON, a member of the Tla-o-qui-aht First Nation, worked for Interior Health as a health lead in the Aboriginal Health Program from 2011 to 2018. After earning her science degree from the University of Victoria, Danielle continued her education and career path in environmental and public health. She worked as an environmental health officer for twelve years with Health Canada, First Nation Inuit Health Branch. During this time, she obtained her master's degree in public health from the University of Waterloo. She was the practitioner co-lead on the Culturally Safe Dementia Care research project and a knowledge user on a Canadian Institutes of Health Research–funded grant on diabetes with the University of British Columbia Okanagan. Danielle has been a regional director (Grey-Bruce region) with the Southwest Ontario Aboriginal Health Access Centre since August 2018.

INDEX

Note: "(f)" after a page number indicates a figure; "(t)" after a page number indicates a table.

healing, 20–21, 93, 95–96, 202, 205

health: disparities, 47, 62, 108, 180, 192; equity/inequity, 4, 11, 103, 109, 129, 239; Indigenous, vii, 62, 72, 125; outcomes, 62, 101, 126; services, 29; status, 43, 47–48, 55, 108; system, 133, 135, 238

health care: access, 29–30, 73, 182; providers, 111, 107–27, 191–92, 239; system, 30, 62–63, 73–74, 121–24, 237

holism, 7, 34, 100, 121, 125

honour, 135, 230

housing, 96, 109, 127(t)

hunting, 19, 92, 101, 182

identity, 68, 90, 101, 202

inclusion, 125, 229

income, 9, 43, 134

Indian, use of term, 12n1

Indian Country, 47–48

Indian Health Service, 46, 182, 188, 192

indigeneity, 62, 241

Indigenous: knowledge, 6, 92, 210; use of term, 12n1; worldviews, 7

Indigenous Syndemic Dementia Model (ISDM), 42, 45, 53–57, 54(f)

intergenerational: knowledge sharing, 6, 201, 211, 220; relationships, 95–97, 102, 224–25

International Indigenous Dementia Research Network, 6, 241

Inuit, use of term, 12n1

Inupiaq, 146–75

Kanienkehaka, viii

knowledge: holders, 115; keepers, 11, 91(t), 215, 227; traditional, 196; translation, 6, 216–17, 227

Knowledge Translation and Exchange (KTE), 6, 235

land, 7, 74, 93, 135, 169

language, 7, 20–21, 64; and assimilation, 64, 201, 205; native, 97–99, 137, 148, 174, 203; second, 147; and translation, 142–44

life course, 34, 91, 103; adulthood, 109, 142, 212; birth, 139, 144; childhood, 50, 80–83, 94, 112; death, 50, 144, 182, 188; later life, 7, 184, 197; youth, 96, 100, 215–30

love, 21, 134, 137, 146, 215

Māori people, 3–4, 133–44

marginalization, 71–72, 88, 126, 184, 239

media, 61–75, 198–99, 207–11, 234

medical professionals, 56, 121, 127(t)

medications, 48, 94, 122, 190

medicine: storytelling as, 9; traditional, 20, 92, 121; Western, 88, 93; wheel, 92–93, 99–103

memory: care, 7–8, 135, 141, 197; loss, 7–8, 88, 94; problems, 94

mental health, 4, 74, 184

methods: discourse analysis, 65–66; evaluation, 10, 218; focus groups, 10, 90, 115, 136, 198; interviews, 10, 90, 108, 136, 219; observation, 90, 102; qualitative, 90, 114, 196, 219; quantitative, 219; questionnaire, 199, 216, 219; sharing circle, 115, 122; storytelling, 9, 95, 196–211

Métis, use of term, 12n1

minority culture, 3, 67, 216

mother, 118, 156, 187

Native: peoples, 50, 55, 148; use of term, 12n1

native language, 97–99, 137, 148, 174, 203

New Zealand, 3, 133–44

nursing, 5, 20, 89, 120, 190

obesity, 27, 53, 87–88, 110, 186

older adults, 184, 199

Ontario, 4, 24, 86

oppression, 11, 181–83

Pākehā (New Zealanders of European descent), 12n5, 136, 143

partnership, 103, 198, 217

patients, 56, 110, 125, 184–89, 237